Social & Public Policy of Alzheimer's Disease in the United States

Robert H. Blank

Social & Public Policy of Alzheimer's Disease in the United States

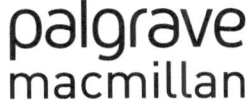

Robert H. Blank
Sarasota, FL, USA

ISBN 978-981-13-0655-6   ISBN 978-981-13-0656-3   (eBook)
https://doi.org/10.1007/978-981-13-0656-3

Library of Congress Control Number: 2018944278

Cover illustration: Pattern adapted from an Indian cotton print produced in the 19th century

Printed on acid-free paper

This Palgrave Pivot imprint is published by the registered company Springer Nature Singapore Pte Ltd. part of Springer Nature.
The registered company address is: 152 Beach Road, #21-01/04 Gateway East, Singapore 189721, Singapore

To Robert M. Sade, MD, and the Institute of Human Values in Health Care at the Medical University of South Carolina

Preface

The inspiration for this book came from an invitation I received to participate in the Pitts Memorial Lectureship in Medical Ethics at the Medical University of South Carolina in April 2017. I was asked to present a public policy perspective on Alzheimer's disease. At the time, I knew little about Alzheimer's, but had written extensively on health and biomedical policy, including three books on brain policy. At the lecture, I learned much about the medical, ethical, social, and other aspects of AD from the other panelists, but it became clear that to date much less attention has been given to the policy dimension.

With further exploration, I found that although there is a huge scientific and social literature and voluminous self-help and narrative books on AD, the literature on public policy is considerably more limited. Recently there have been many extensive commission and government reports, including thorough studies from various AD associations, that include the political and social aspects and provide excellent sources for information and data, but they tend to be unwieldy. This book attempts to fill this void and provide a readable overview of the social policy issues of AD and other dementias. It synthesizes perspectives on wide range of issues raised by AD as reflected in research funding, professional association reports and guidelines, commission reports, regulations, and laws.

Because of my long-standing interest in cross-national policy, I feel that it is crucial to include the policies of countries other than the United States. Although much of the current published AD policy work has a US/European focus, recently there has been increasing activity on the global impact of AD that underscores the considerable variation among countries as to how proactive they have been in dealing with it as well as widespread differences in the perception of AD and how best to treat affected individuals. Therefore, although this book concentrates on the public policy and political aspects of AD in the United States, it includes some coverage of the global dimensions and AD policies in other countries where appropriate.

Sarasota, FL, USA   Robert H. Blank

CONTENTS

About the Author

Robert H. Blank, PhD (University of Maryland), is Adjunct Professor of Political Science at the University of Canterbury in Christchurch, New Zealand, and a research scholar at New College of Florida. He has been a frequent guest professor at Aarhus University in Denmark and at National Taiwan University in Taipei, Taiwan. His previous academic positions include Chair of Public Policy at Brunel University in West London, Professor and Associate Director of the Program for Biosocial Research at Northern Illinois University, and Chair of Political Science at the University of Idaho. He has held residential fellowships at Vanderbilt University, Stanford University, Indiana University, and the Medical University of South Carolina, and Fulbright Lectureships in Taiwan (1976–1977 and 2007) and New Zealand (1984). He has taught, lectured, and written widely in the areas of comparative health policy, medical technology assessment, genetic and reproductive policy, and neuroscience policy. Among the many books he has written are *Rationing Medicine, Regulating Reproduction, Brain Policy, The Price of Life, Biology and Political Science, Comparative Health Policy,* 1st–5th editions, *End of Life Decision Making: A Comparative Study, Condition Critical, Governing Home Care, Intervention in the Brain: Politics and Policy,* and *Cognitive Enhancement.* He was co-editor of *The Palgrave International Handbook of Healthcare Policy and Governance.*

CHAPTER 1

Alzheimer's Disease and Other Dementias: An Introduction

Abstract This chapter first discusses the definition of Alzheimer's disease (AD) and distinguishes it from other dementias. It illustrates how problematic it is to diagnose it precisely, in part because it is often mixed with other types, but also because it can vary among individuals. The chapter next examines the stages of AD and the accompanying symptoms at each stage. It then turns attention to competing theories of the causes of AD and to the range of frameworks for studying it. Although the disease model is predominant in the literature, it is not without controversy. The chapter then summarizes testing possibilities for AD, other forms of cognitive impairment, and asymptomatic individuals at high risk of developing AD. Finally, it presents data on AD prevalence and deaths in the United States and at the global level.

Keywords Alzheimer's disease (AD) • Dementia • Mini Mental State Examination (MMSE) • Stages of Alzheimer's • Symptoms of Alzheimer's

This chapter first discusses the definition of Alzheimer's disease (AD) and distinguishes it from other dementias. It illustrates how problematic it is to diagnose, in part because it is often mixed with other types, but also because it varies among individuals. The chapter next examines the stages of AD and the symptoms at each stage. It then turns attention to competing theories of the causes of AD and to the range of frameworks for studying it. Although the disease model is predominant in the literature, it remains highly controversial. The chapter then analyzes testing possibilities for AD, other forms of cognitive impairment, and asymptomatic individuals at high risk of developing AD. Finally, it presents data on AD prevalence and deaths in the United States and globally.

DEFINING ALZHEIMER'S DISEASE AND OTHER DEMENTIAS

AD is a progressive and irreversible brain disorder which gradually damages a person's memory, judgment, reasoning skills, personality, autonomy, and, ultimately, bodily functions. Although the cause remains unknown, it results in a measured loss of neurons, damage to neurons so they no longer function properly, and a loss of synapses (neural connections) through which messages are passed from neuron to neuron. Also known as late-onset Alzheimer's disease, AD is primarily a disease of older adults, although the first noticeable symptoms can occur much earlier. Early-onset AD (EAD) sometimes can affect people as young as 30 but this is rare. When AD runs in families, it is called familial Alzheimer's disease (FAD). The underlying causes and specific risk factors for AD remain unclear despite considerable research investment.

In 2011, the National Institute on Aging (NIA) and the Alzheimer's Association (AA) proposed revised criteria and guidelines for diagnosing AD. These criteria and guidelines update those published in 1984 by the National Institute of Neurological Disorders and Stroke and the AA. The criteria of the earlier version were based chiefly on a doctor's clinical judgment about the cause of an individual's symptoms as described by the individual and family members, the results of cognitive tests, and a general neurological assessment. The new criteria incorporate three notable changes. First, they identify two stages of AD: mild cognitive impairment (MCI) due to AD and dementia due to AD. This contrasts with the earlier criteria where dementia was already apparent. Second, they propose for research purposes criteria for a pre-clinical phase before symptoms such as memory loss develop. And third, they incorporate biomarker tests that can indicate the presence or absence of AD, or the risk of developing it. Although finding a simple and inexpensive test, such as a blood test, would be ideal for patients and physicians, to date no test has shown the accuracy and reliability needed to diagnose AD based on that criterion alone.

MCI is a condition in which a person has mild but measurable changes in thinking abilities that are noticeable to oneself and close others, but do not affect the capacity for everyday activities. Approximately 15–20 percent of people aged 65 or older have MCI. People with MCI, especially that involving memory problems, are more likely to develop AD than those without it. A recent review found that 32 percent of individuals with MCI developed AD within five years (Ward et al. 2013). Identifying which individuals with MCI are most likely to develop AD is a major research goal, according to Livingston et al. (2017).

Similarly, in 1988, the National Institute of Neurological and Communicative Disorders and Stroke and the Alzheimer's and Related Disorders Association defined three diagnostic categories: possible, probable, and definite AD. Definite AD can be confirmed only at autopsy after a brain biopsy confirms the presence of characteristic neurofibrillary tangles. Probable AD is diagnosed clinically when the patient meets core clinical criteria which can be supplemented by tests, including cerebrospinal fluid levels of tau protein or beta-amyloid precursor protein (Alonso Vilatela et al. 2012). In 2012, the NIA and the AA developed guidelines to help pathologists describe and categorize the brain changes associated with AD and other dementias on autopsy.

The Mini Mental State Examination (MMSE) is the most commonly used test to help clinicians diagnose AD and to assess its progression and severity. The MMSE tests numerous mental abilities, including a person's memory, attention, and language. Clinicians consider a person's score along with their history, symptoms, a physical exam, and the results of other tests including brain scans. The MMSE can also be used to assess changes in a person who has already been diagnosed with AD and help clarify how severe a person's symptoms are and how quickly they are progressing (see Box 1.1). Some commentators have been critical of the current diagnostic criteria. For instance, Sabat (2018) contends that while the conventional formulaic questionnaire (usually MMSE) is useful in medical diagnostics, it is vulnerable to the pitfalls of stereotyping and labeling. For Sabat it is important to understand the subjective experience of AD: how does the person react to those losses imposed by AD, how do caregivers react, and what do their reactions mean to the person diagnosed? In an extensive review of cognitive screening trials by the US Preventive Services Task Force, Lin et al. (2013) found no trial that examined the effect of screening on patient, caregiver, or clinician decision making or important individual or societal outcomes.

Box 1.1 Cognitive Quotients (QuoCo)
The MMSE continues to be used to screen for cognitive impairment, but it remains unclear how to interpret changes in its score over time to distinguish age associated-cognitive decline from early degenerative process. To rectify this, Canadian researchers devised a tool, the QuoCo, to enable doctors to track an individual's cognitive performance over time (Bernier et al. 2017). They found that QuoCo was 80 percent accurate in identifying those with dementia and 89 percent for those without it. Although QuoCo constitutes only part of diagnostic process and must be interpreted by a physician with a full clinical history and physical examination to eliminate other causes of cognitive changes, it offers a longitudinal evaluation to facilitate initiation of further investigation and treatment when appropriate.

The Diagnostic and Statistical Manual of Mental Disorders (DSM-5) stopped using the word "dementia" and instead uses the phrase "major neurocognitive disorders," or illnesses with demonstrable neural substrate abnormalities together with cognitive symptoms that occur in people who have had normal brain development (Sachdev et al. 2014). In some cases, individuals with symptoms of dementia do not actually have it, but rather a condition that mimics those of dementia. Causes of dementia-like symptoms can include depression, medication side effects, thyroid problems, certain vitamin deficiencies, and alcohol abuse, many of which can be mitigated with treatment. Medication side effects are especially prominent among older people prescribed multiple drugs for chronic physical conditions. One study reported that 9 percent of people with dementia-like symptoms had other conditions that were potentially reversible (Clarfield 2003).

AD is the most common form of dementia, constituting an estimated 60–80 percent. Symptoms vary among individuals, but the most common initial symptom is a worsening ability to remember new information. This happens because the first neurons to be damaged and destroyed with AD are those in brain regions involved in forming new memories. As neurons in other parts of the brain are destroyed, broader cognitive and functional abilities deteriorate. The pace at which symptoms advance from mild to moderate to severe varies from person to person. The characteristic pathologies of AD are the progressive accumulation of the protein fragment beta-amyloid (plaques) outside neurons in the brain, twisted strands of the protein tau (tangles) inside neurons, lesions of cholinergic neurons together with synaptic alterations in cerebral cortex, hippocampus, and other brain regions, eventually accompanied by the damage and death of neurons (Wu et al. 2011).

Vascular dementia (VD), previously known as multi-infarct or post-stroke dementia, as a sole cause of dementia accounts for about 10 percent, but around 50 percent of AD patients also display pathologic evidence of vascular dementia (see Bowler and Hachinski 2003). Unlike the memory loss associated with AD, the initial symptoms of VD are more likely to be impaired judgment or inability to make decisions, plan, or organize. People with VD also often have difficulty with motor function, particularly slow gait and poor balance. VD commonly follows blood vessel blockage or damage from strokes or bleeding in the brain. The location, number, and size of the brain injuries determine whether dementia will follow and how much the individual's thinking and physical functioning will be affected.

Parkinson's disease (PD) is most associated with early problems with movement including slowness, rigidity, tremor, and changes in gait. In PD, alpha-synuclein aggregates appear deep in the brain in the substantia nigra. These aggregates are thought to cause degeneration of the nerve cells that produce dopamine. The incidence of PD is about one-tenth that of AD. As PD progresses, it often produces dementia secondary to the accumulation of Lewy bodies in the cortex or the accumulation of beta-amyloid clumps and tau tangles like that of found in AD.

Dementia with Lewy bodies (DLB) shares some symptoms with AD, but early sufferers are more likely to have sleep disturbances, visual hallucinations, slowness, gait imbalance, or other Parkinsonian movement features, as well as visuospatial impairment, that may occur before significant memory impairment. Lewy bodies are abnormal aggregations of the protein alpha-synuclein in neurons. When they develop in the cortex, dementia can result. Although people with DLB and PD both have Lewy bodies, the onset of PD is marked by motor impairment and LBD by cognitive impairment.

Frontotemporal lobar degeneration (FTLD) includes dementias such as behavioral-variant FTLD, primary progressive aphasia, Pick's disease, cortico-basal degeneration, and progressive supranuclear palsy that collectively account for under 10 percent of dementia cases. Typical early symptoms include marked changes in personality and behavior and/or difficulty producing or comprehending language. Unlike AD, memory is normally spared in the initial stages and most people develop symptoms at a younger age, generally 45–60.

Mixed dementia is characterized by the hallmark abnormalities of more than one cause of dementia. Most commonly this constitutes AD combined with VD, followed by AD with DLB, and AD with both VD and DLB. Vascular dementia with DLB is much less common. Recent studies suggest that mixed dementia is more common than previously recognized, with about half of older people with AD having pathologic evidence of more than one cause. These studies also show that the likelihood of having mixed dementia increases with age and is highest in those aged 85 or older. To acknowledge the increasing recognition of mixed dementia, the National Academies of Sciences, Engineering, and Medicine (NASEM) (2017) uses the term clinical Alzheimer's-type dementia (CATD) instead of AD (see Box 1.2).

Box 1.2 NASEM Categories of Cognitive Impairment

Age-related cognitive decline (ARCD): Deterioration in cognitive performance that is a normal part of aging. It is also sometimes referred to as cognitive aging. *Mild cognitive impairment (MCI)*: Cognitive impairment that has reached a level of deterioration from normal cognitive function identifiable by individuals, family members, or clinicians, but without significant functional impairment in daily activities. *Clinical Alzheimer's-type dementia (CATD)*: Cognitive impairment severe enough that an individual can no longer function independently. This term is not widely used in the field; the committee uses it here to reflect the increasing recognition of mixed dementia, which may be difficult to differentiate in a clinical setting.

There has been serious concern raised over the "Alzheimerization" of dementia or the widespread perception, especially in the United States, that AD is the most significant and research-worthy type of dementia. This term refers not only to the unbalanced funding focus on AD but also to the concentration of cultural and academic attention accorded to AD to the detriment of other types (Hodgson 2011). Furthermore, dementia criteria are largely modeled on those of AD. This is a problem for other dementias, particularly vascular and Lewy body where memory impairment is not the chief early manifestation, thus leading to missed opportunities for prevention or treatment (Abou-Saleh et al. 2011). According to Howard (2005), Alzheimerization of dementia diagnosis has become so dominant that clinicians are missing cases where the control of vascular risk factors is more helpful than prescription of a cholinesterase inhibitor. In sum, it has stacked the deck against making a diagnosis of anything other than AD. Fukui (2016) agrees that it is an obstruction to the diagnosis of non-AD-type dementia and argues that a neuropsychological bottom-up approach to symptoms of dementia could minimize the problem. As noted by the Lewy Body Dementia Association, "Those of us in the LBD community are aware that Alzheimer's is just one type of dementia… but, unfortunately, most news outlets use the term 'Alzheimer's' when they should be using 'dementia' " (https://www.lbda.org/sites/default/files/media).

Although it is important to reiterate that AD is but one of the many forms of dementia and that each type has different manifestations and causes, for readability the term AD is used here. In those instances where other forms of cognitive impairment are discussed, or the data refers to dementia in the more inclusive sense, the term "dementia" is used. Also, again for clarity, the term "AD patient" rather than "person with Alzheimer's" is often used to refer to anyone diagnosed with it, even though some commentators object to the use of the term "patient" for reasons discussed later.

STAGES OF ALZHEIMER'S DISEASE

Although the progression of AD is a continuum and varies by individual, normally it is viewed as having three distinct stages. The early, or mild, stage of AD is often discounted by relatives, friends, and sometimes professionals who see it as just a normal part of aging. Because the onset of the disease is gradual, it is difficult to be sure exactly when it begins. Early symptoms can include: becoming forgetful, especially of things that just occurred; some difficulty with communication, such as finding appropriate words; becoming disoriented in familiar places; losing track of the time; difficulty making decisions and handling personal finances; diminished judgment; losing things and blaming others; loss of interest in normal activities; and changes in personality with increased irritability, depression or anxiety, or occasional anger outbursts.

As the disease progresses to the intermediate, or middle, stage, these problems become more apparent, consistent, and restricting and include: becoming very forgetful, especially of recent events and people's names and faces; difficulty comprehending time, date, and place and confusing past events with the present; increasing difficulty with speech and comprehension; inability to live alone safely without considerable support; behavioral changes that may include wandering, repeated questioning, calling out, clinging, hallucinations, and aggression.

The final, or late, stage is one of nearly total dependence and inactivity with a need for continuous care. Memory disturbances become very serious and the physical side of the disease becomes obvious. At this stage, the patient: is usually unaware of time and place; has difficulty understanding what is happening around him or her; is unable to recognize relatives, friends, and once-familiar objects; is unable to eat without assistance and might have difficulty swallowing; needs assisted self-care for bathing and toileting; might have bladder and bowel incontinence; might be unable to walk or be confined to a wheelchair or bed; and might have escalating behavioral problems including aggression and non-verbal agitation such as kicking, hitting, screaming, or moaning. Often the symptoms worsen at night with an inability to sleep. At the end stage, ventilators or other mechanical support will be needed for life support, without which death will result.

Theories on the Causes of Alzheimer's Disease

According to a recent Lancet Commission, despite impressive research efforts over the past three decades, the causal mechanisms of AD remain unclear (Winblad et al. 2016). This has led to an array of variant theories on the causes of AD, some of which have been predominant at various times. It is quite likely that multiple theories are involved.

The Cholinergic Hypothesis

The systematic biochemical investigation of the brains of patients with AD began in the late 1960s and early 1970s. The hope was that a clearly defined neurochemical abnormality would be identified, providing the basis for the development of therapeutic interventions. The cholinergic hypothesis focused on neurotransmitters, their receptors, and neural circuits and claimed that acetylcholine, especially nicotinic cholinergic systems, was important for memory and attention. It posited that degeneration of cholinergic neurons in the basal forebrain and the associated loss of cholinergic neurotransmission in the cerebral cortex and other areas contributed significantly to the deterioration in cognitive function seen in patients with AD (Bartus et al. 1982). However, after 20 years of dominance, evidence from numerous studies challenged the cholinergic theory's veracity as an explanation for AD and it lost favor by the mid-1990s (Francis et al. 1999).

Amyloid Cascade Hypothesis

When medical science in general moved from a systems neuroscience perspective to genetics and molecular biology, an opening emerged to replace the cholinergic hypothesis with one that was assumed to be more powerful, that is, the amyloid cascade hypothesis. This theory proposes that excessive accumulation of a peptide called beta-amyloid in the brain disrupts communication among brain cells, eventually killing them, thus causing AD. When a large protein called amyloid precursor protein (APP) is activated, it is cut by other proteins into separate, smaller sections, and, under certain circumstances, one of the fragments produced is beta-amyloid. Because it is chemically "stickier" than other fragments, it accumulates in stages, first forming small clusters called oligomers, then chains of clusters called fibrils, then mats of fibrils called beta-sheets. The final stage is beta-amyloid plaques, which contain clumps of beta-sheets and other substances, that are considered a characteristic of a brain affected by AD. According to the amyloid cascade hypothesis, these stages of beta-amyloid aggregation disrupt cell-to-cell communication and activate immune cells. These immune cells, in turn, trigger inflammation, ultimately destroying the brain cells and causing dementia (Alzheimer's Association 2017).

Despite capturing the bulk of research funding, not all scientists believe that beta-amyloid is the primary cause of AD. Although there are several lines of evidence that support this theory, there are numerous challenges to it. For one thing, the beta-amyloid that accumulates in plaques occurs in normal aging as well as AD. Approximately 30 percent of people without any signs of dementia have brains replete with beta-amyloid at autopsy (Luan et al. 2013). Some people's brains appear to be more resilient to plaques than others and their existence does not mean they will exhibit AD in their lifetime. In addition, the alleged cascade from amyloid accumulation to cell death to clinical dementia includes many hypothetical steps that may not occur at all in all cases and certainly not in a linear fashion (Whitehouse 2014). The association between the amyloid plaque formation and neurofibrillary tangles, which seem more closely related to neuronal dysfunction and death, is also unclear. Moreover, we do not understand how or even if beta-amyloid kills neurons. They could, instead, be the brain's attempt to dispatch repair mechanisms and compensate for impaired structure or function, thus efforts to lower amyloid production or removal of deposited amyloid could in fact exacerbate the disease process (Whitehouse 2014). Finally, despite billions of dollars spent over two decades on the basic biology and extensive clinical trials that focused on therapies and vaccines to modify the amyloid cascade, there has not yet been an effective therapy.

The Tau Hypothesis

These problems with the amyloid hypothesis have led many in the AD field to ask whether a second misfolded protein, tau, is the real driver of the condition's neurodegeneration and symptoms. The tau hypothesis states that excessive or abnormal phosphorylation of tau results in the transformation of normal adult tau into paired helical filament tau (PHF-tau) and neurofibrillary tangles (NFTs) that form inside dying cells. Tangles are twisted fibers that destroy a vital cell transport system made of proteins. Normally, tau helps keep the transport system on track, but in areas where tangles are forming, the twisted strands of tau essentially disintegrate the transport system so that nutrients and other essential supplies can no longer move through the cells, which eventually die. Recently, researchers developed PET imaging agents that can bind to tau in the living brain. When they measured tau in the study participants' cerebral spinal fluid (CSF), higher levels were correlated with increased tau in the temporal lobe, a region involved in memory processing. Tau has been found to be a sounder predictor of when people transition from the early, pre-symptomatic stages of the disease into mild AD (Brier et al. 2016).

One conclusion is that the cumulative insults from beta-amyloid and tau drive the decline in cognition. Although the brain may be able to compensate for the deficits caused by beta-amyloid, once tau tangles start to spread, the brain loses its capacity do so. Although most people develop some plaques and tangles as they age, those with AD tend to have far more of both. Moreover, the plaques and tangles tend to form in a predictable pattern, beginning in areas important in learning and memory and then spreading to other regions of the brain.

Other Theories of AD

Although these two dominant theories are now the most extensively discussed, due to their failure to explain the causes adequately, other theories have proliferated. For instance, the anti-oxidant theory holds that free radicals (atoms with at least one unpaired electron that are unstable and weekly bonded) accumulate in the brain and damage nerve cells by altering their chemical structure, thereby triggering disruptions that result in loss of cell function. It posits that free-radical damage can accelerate the progression of cancer, heart disease, and age-related degenerative diseases including AD. Clinical trials of anti-oxidants like vitamin E or diets rich in anti-oxidant-rich fruits and vegetables assumed to neutralize free radicals by donating their electrons for stability, however, have been disappointing.

Another theory is the inflammatory theory which posits that deleterious molecules often associated with senile plaques are triggered by infections or traumatic head injuries by transforming beta-amyloid proteins and causing them to form insoluble plaques. However, the use of nonsteroidal anti-inflammatory drugs (NSAIDs) to suppress this process has not been successful. Similarly, the infectious disease hypothesis suggests that AD is caused by slow viruses known as prions that are made of proteins rather than DNA or RNA. However, while some herpes viruses and other infectious diseases can produce dementia, they are not consistently related to AD. Other theories include the excitatory cell death hypothesis where excess firing of neurotransmitters like glutamate could cause neurons to fire, or excite, themselves to death, and the AD–diabetes hypothesis based on a link between glucose metabolism and dementia characterized by progressive insulin deficiency and insulin resistance. Although scientific support for many of these theories is wanting, this has not stopped biomedical entrepreneurs from exploiting them (see Chap. 3).

As noted above, many older people exhibit mixed dementias in which the cognitive disabilities present in late age could be a function of many factors acting over a lifetime, including environmental factors such as toxins. It seems reasonable, therefore, not to conclude that one hypothesis is specious and another explanatory, but rather that many theories might have an element of veracity. Therefore, studies of potential multiple causes of dementia and the cumulative or synergistic effects of many contributing factors are in order given the failure the favored theories thus far.

Frameworks of Alzheimer's Disease

Although the literature on AD tends to focus on disease/medical models, more holistic conceptualizations as explicated in much social science literature are emerging. Innes (2009), for instance, unpacks AD from different disciplines, including biomedical approaches that focus on cognitive functioning, psychosocial approaches that focus on personhood and person-centered care, and social-gerontological approaches that examine how AD is socially constructed. Another approach is the public health model which shifts attention to prevention and health promotion strategies. According to Whitehouse (2014), we must recalibrate the study of AD from an almost exclusive focus on biochemical, molecular pharmacological, and genetic aspects to include ecological and psychosocial models of health. His term "ecopsychosociology" expands the biopsychosocial model of health to encompass ecology as a dominant form of biological thinking in relationship to disease.

A provocative perspective on AD is that it is nothing but normal aging and, since we cannot cure aging, we need an enlightened view of AD and what it means to be an aging human. For Whitehouse and George (2008) AD is a myth, based on hype and false hope, perpetuated by a powerful research community and the pharmaceutical industry. AD does not "claim as victims" older people, but rather simply alters how one lives his or her life. It is not a singular disease that can be differentiated from normal aging and there is no evidence it is an "epidemic" other than the fact there are more people living to old age. Moreover, it is an illusion that science will one day win the war against AD, because that would require halting the natural process of brain aging. They contend that an unfortunate consequence of this myth is that many people suffer from an overwhelming fear of a decline in the ability to store and recall memories rather than view it as part of an aging process brought on by a variety of factors. All humans to some degree gradually lose vision, hearing, sense of smell, and, also, memory. Thus, dementia is best seen as a continuum along which we all progress at different rates. In our attempt to make sense of a natural process that we cannot control, we have created an antagonist—a terrorizing disease of the brain called AD that scientists can fight against—but, in fact, the talk of a cure is based on faith, not scientific extrapolations. According to Whitehouse (2014) we need to liberate ourselves from the "tyranny" of the AD medical narrative and create a new framework for brain aging from one of a disease to one of a life-long process fraught with challenges. Instead of treating them as diseased, we should view them as aging humans presenting the human condition.

Like Whitehead, Power (2010) argues that dementia care in this country is medicalized rather than humanized and that a cultural reassessment is necessary. He advocates a comprehensive transformation in the way society and particularly medical and societal institutions treat individuals with AD. If it was viewed not as a neuropathology, but rather as a different way of perceiving the world, personhood could be restored. Power embraces models of what he terms "experiential" institutional care that relies less on drug therapy and routine and more on personalized care and individual autonomy (see Chap. 4 discussion on social health). Just as Power emphasizes the need for a paradigm shift in how we perceive AD, Kosik and Clegg (2010) advocate a shift in the way we treat the disease. They contend that to avoid bankrupting the nation and to better serve the needs of the individuals caught up in the disease the emerging crisis in demographics necessitates a major shift in health care policy away from medicalization of AD.

According to Genova (2008), however, proclaiming that AD is not a disease, but just a normal part of aging, as Whitehead does, is "plainly wrong and irresponsible." Normal aging is forgetting someone's name, but AD is forgetting your spouse's name. Convincing people that AD is not a disease and should not be diagnosed (or labeled as Whitehouse terms it) will needlessly keep people who are suffering with AD away from doctors, treatment options, and planning responsibly for their future. Although many of the points the critics of the medical model of AD make are valuable for a policy debate, this book presumes that there is, in fact, an Alzheimer's disease and that efforts to find its cause and treat it are warranted. At the same time, policy makers must consider a broad range of approaches in making policies that are best for persons with dementia, their caregivers, and society.

TESTING FOR AD, MCI, AND PRE-DEMENTIA

The emerging awareness, and fear, of AD and the movement of baby boomers into late middle age, accompanied by their experience of seeing aging parents with AD and concerns for themselves, have led to an increased demand for earlier diagnoses and pre-symptomatic testing to determine one's risk for developing it. Recent advances in genetics, biomarkers, and neuroimaging have an increasing potential to meet these emerging demands (Alzheimer's Association 2016). Simultaneously, the designation of a pre-dementia diagnosis, that is, MCI, and the successful marketing of DNA testing have produced an environment in which people want to know their genetic health status.

AD can be associated with a family history (40 percent of patients with AD have at least one other afflicted first-degree relative) or it can be idiopathic. Between 1995 and 2009, more than 500 potential new susceptibility genes were reported, but none of them have been consistently replicated and confirmed (Winblad et al. 2016). In their comprehensive analysis of the genetics of AD, Alonso Vilatela et al. (2012) estimate that the amount of risk of AD attributable to genetics is around 70 percent, although others place it lower. Over 100 genes, particularly on chromosomes 9, 10, and 12, have been associated with late-onset AD; while mutations in chromosomes 1, 14, and 21 have been associated with FAD. Genetic testing for early-onset FAD is clinically available for PSEN1, PSEN2, and APP mutations in clinical laboratories and has been investigated both in patients with probable AD and in asymptomatic family members.

However, at present for most persons with AD, there is no reliable genetic predictor. Although those with one copy of the apolipoprotein E epsilon 4 allele (ApoE-e4) have a two to five times risk of having AD compared to those who do not carry the gene, the positive predictive value of this testing in the general population is low, and consensus conferences have been uniform in stating that predictive genetic testing is insufficiently accurate for pre-symptomatic testing (Hayden 2008). Despite the current limitations in knowledge, however, genetics is certain to play a major part in understanding the mechanisms of AD and will have an important role in future implementation of prevention and care strategies (Winblad et al. 2016).

Recent developments in biological markers for AD are more encouraging. Several diagnostic biomarkers have been developed to detect AD neuropathology even in individuals in pre-clinical stages (Box 1.3). "Diagnostic biomarkers" are markers of in vivo pathology that are present at all stages of the disease, and, therefore, can be used to detect AD pathological changes in the asymptomatic state. By contrast, "progression markers," which might have poor disease specificity for use at early stages, can trace changes as AD progresses. Amyloid imaging and CSF biomarkers enable early detection of AD and, importantly, discernment of patients with MCI who have underlying pathology that puts them at a high risk of progression to AD dementia (Lerner 2013). Other biomarkers measure levels of total tau protein and other proteins in the blood.

> **Box 1.3 Blood Test for Amyloid-β Protein Buildup**
> Researchers in Japan and Australia recently developed a blood test to detect amyloid-β protein accumulation in the brain (Nakamura et al. 2018). Using immunoprecipitation and mass spectrometry, the team isolated and characterized amyloid proteins in the blood from a cohort of 121 subjects in Japan, and a validation cohort of 252 in Australia, spanning a range of cognitive function from normal to developed AD. They found that all test biomarkers, especially the composite, showed high performance when predicting brain amyloid-β burden and that the blood tests could predict amyloid-β levels with about 90 percent of the accuracy achieved using PET scanning. The authors note that these plasma biomarkers have cost and scalability advantages over current techniques, enabling broader clinical access and efficient population screening.

Recently, the Geneva Task Force for the Roadmap of Alzheimer's Biomarkers was established to deliver a systematic strategic research agenda to promote effective validation of AD biomarkers and to foster their use in clinical practice (Porteri et al. 2017). Moreover, the advent of technical advances such as exome sequencing (reading the sequence of the coding regions of every gene in one test) and whole genome sequencing (reading the entire sequence for the human genome in one test) is transforming the process of genetic testing by sequencing numerous genes simultaneously for the same cost of what it cost for several genes with previous technologies (Loy et al. 2014).

Biomarkers of functional impairment, neuronal loss, and protein deposition that can be assessed by MRI or PET neuroimaging or CSF analysis are increasingly being used to diagnose AD in research studies and specialist clinical settings. For instance, recent advances in imaging amyloid in the human brain using PET have reinforced efforts to identify biomarkers to diagnose the disease and monitor therapy (Villemagne et al. 2012). However, the validation of the clinical usefulness of these biomarkers is incomplete, which is hindering reimbursement by health insurance providers and their widespread clinical implementation (Frisoni et al. 2017).

Moreover, the Centers for Medicare and Medicaid Services, which is responsible for reimbursement decisions, has, despite Food and Drug Administration (FDA) approval, declined to pay for amyloid imaging except under very limited clinical trial circumstances.

Despite mounting interest in AD biomarkers, their inclusion in clinical criteria raises ethical and social issues concerning the reactions of those who undergo pre-symptomatic diagnoses and MCI testing. Asymptomatic individuals who want to know whether they are susceptible to AD can now arrange for predictive testing, even though the tests are far from fail-safe. Furthermore, even if testing demonstrates a risk, the times from onset of symptoms and decline to a dependent state are unpredictable. Therefore, when researchers recently announced a blood test for AD, reactions were mixed. Most experts welcomed the news, but others worried that, until effective treatments are available, learning that you are likely to develop AD could cause more harm than good. On the plus side, such a test can permit more effective early treatment and motivate people who learn that they are at heightened risk to make healthy lifestyle changes. Additionally, early detection can allow people to make informed decisions about their care before the symptoms of AD become obstructive—one reason both the AA and the Alzheimer's Foundation of America support early diagnosis. Moreover, a negative test could relieve a person from the anxiety of developing AD (Baum 2016).

On the negative side, a positive finding could change a person's outlook on life, making him or her even more anxious, depressed, withdrawn, and ashamed. One study found that those who learned they tested positive judged their memories more critically and performed worse on memory tests than those who were not told (Jaret 2014). Thus, the stress of learning that you are at high risk to develop AD could worsen the symptoms of forgetfulness and confusion. Stites and associates (2017) found that persons with MCI or AD who were made aware of their diagnosis reported lower average satisfaction with daily life, basic functioning, and physical wellbeing, and experienced more difficulties in daily life than those who were unaware, independent of the severity of cognitive impairment. Moreover, those expecting their condition to worsen over time reported greater depression, higher stress, lower quality of daily life, and more cognitive difficulties compared to those oblivious of these facts about themselves.

Apprehension is directed especially toward direct-to-consumer kits that are readily available commercially and allow wide-scale biotesting without medical advice or counseling. Furthermore, despite often dramatic headlines announcing a new blood test for AD, for example "Alzheimer's disease could be prevented after new blood test breakthrough," it is not as imminent or promising as one author exclaimed: "A blood test has been developed to predict if someone will develop Alzheimer's within a year, raising hopes that the disease could become preventable... The blood test, which could be available in as little as two years, was described as a 'major step forward' by Jeremy Hunt, the Health Secretary, and by charities which said it could revolutionize research into a cure" (Knapton 2014: 1). Other scientists caution that the results must be replicated in other laboratories and that the researchers are overly optimistic about the clinical benefit of the test, at least so far. One commentator observed that if the study cohort's 5 percent rate of conversion from normal cognition to mild impairment or AD is representative of a real-world screening population, the test would have a positive predictive value of just 35 percent, meaning that nearly two-thirds of positive screening results would be false (Lab Tests Online 2014).

Tests for AD also raise concerns about possible adverse selection in insurance markets by people who buy long-term insurance once they receive a positive finding. To test this, Zick et al. (2005) followed 148 cognitively normal people participating in a randomized clinical trial of genetic testing for AD for one year after risk assessment and ApoE-e4 genotype disclosure. Although they found no significant differences for health, life, or disability insurance purchases, those who tested positive were 5.76 times more likely to have augmented their long-term care insurance than those who did not. If genetic testing for AD risk assessment becomes common, it could trigger adverse selection in long-term care insurance.

Despite recent advances in testing, the BlueCross BlueShield Association Technology Evaluation Center Assessment concluded that there are insufficient studies to indicate that ApoE genotyping provides sufficient sensitivity or specificity to allow it to be used as a diagnostic test in symptomatic individuals. Based on the lack of peer-reviewed literature, testing for AD is considered investigational and, thus, denied coverage by Blue Cross/Blue Shield (BCBS 2016). The sensitivity and specificity of genetic testing for indicating which individuals will progress to AD is low, and numerous other factors can affect progression. Moreover, there is no evidence to indicate that genetic testing would change the medical management of the symptomatic patient to improve outcomes. The Joint Practice Guidelines of the American College of Genetics and the National Society of Genetic Counsellors recommend against pediatric testing for AD. Direct-to-consumer testing is not advised and at least a three-generation family history should be obtained with specific information regarding diagnosis of AD in affected family members.

Despite these caveats, a growing number of companies are marketing general DNA or specific tests for AD. Although some sites disclose the scientific limits of their tests, other do not. One example is:

True Health Lab—Regular price $529 but sale at $299.

Spectracell collection locations:

1. Free draw at Any Lab Test Now!
2. Or you can contact your local hospital, clinic, or phlebotomy service. Inform them that you have a test kit that requires a draw. They do not need to know who Spectracell nor True Health Labs are. Nominal draw fees may apply. http://www.truehealthlabs.com/Apolipoprotein-E-APOE-Test-p/SpectraCell_Apo_E.htm.

Also see: https://labtestsonline.org/news/140326alzheimer/ and http://www.insightpharmareports.com/Affiliated-Reports/Global-Data/PharmaFocus—Biomarkers-in-Alzheimer-s-Disease/.

In the end, government regulation will play a major role in biomarker development, clinical market access, and use in drug discovery in both the United States and EU (PharmaFocus 2013).

Prevalence and Deaths Attributed to AD in the United States

The prevalence of AD varies considerably by age group, with 4 percent under age 65, 15 percent aged 65–74, 44 percent aged 75–84, and 37 percent aged over 85 years. Starting at age 65, the risk of developing AD doubles every five years. By age 85, between 25 percent and 50 percent will exhibit signs of AD (Sinclair 2016). In 2018, an estimated 5.7 million Americans had AD, 81 percent of whom were aged 75 or older (Alzheimer's Association 2018). When the first wave of baby boomers reaches age 85 in 2031, it is projected that more than three million will have AD. Approximately 476,000 people aged 65 or older developed AD in the United States in 2017: 63,000 new cases were from 65 to 74, 172,000 were from 75 to 84, and 241,000 were aged 85 and older. Moreover, by 2050 the oldest-old are expected to increase from 14 to 22 percent of those aged 65 and older. Because of this, the annual number of new cases of AD is projected to double to almost one million by 2050. Barring the development of medical breakthroughs to prevent or cure AD, by 2050 the number of people aged 65 and older with AD is expected to nearly triple, from 5.2 million to 13.8 million, although previous estimates based on high-range projections of population growth provided by the US Census suggest that this number may be as high as 16 million (Hurd et al. 2013).

A continuing difficulty is procuring accurate data on AD deaths. When a person dies, the cause or causes of death are listed on death certificates and filed with each state's Bureau of Vital Statistics. This information is then forwarded to the National Center for Health Statistics of the Centers for Disease Control and Prevention (CDC), which compiles and reports the totals each year as the official US mortality figures and leading causes of death. Based on this process, AD is often listed as the sixth leading cause of death in the United States, but recent evidence suggests that deaths from AD are five to six times higher than reported by the CDC, and that it is the third leading cause. Underreporting of AD as a cause of death on death certificates is a well-known phenomenon because some people with AD never receive a diagnosis while many others have dementia-related conditions, such as aspiration pneumonia, listed as the primary cause of death.

Two groups of investigators examined this to discover the full burden of AD. While their estimates of deaths due to AD vary slightly, both groups determined that AD-related mortality rates are significantly higher than the official figure. In one study, the researchers combined data from the Chicago Health and Aging Project with US Census data to estimate the number of deaths of older Americans with AD (Weuve et al. 2014). After computing age-, sex-, race-, and education-specific AD incidences and education-adjusted AD mortality proportions specific to these groups, they combined these probabilities with US-wide census, education, and mortality data. They found that an estimated 600,000 people aged 65 and older with AD died in 2010 compared to the CDC's 83,494 figure. Moreover, they estimate that this number will rise to 900,000 in 2030 and to 1.6 million by 2050.

Similarly, the second study, based on autopsy findings, found that the number of deaths due to AD in people 75 and older could be six times higher than the official count (James et al. 2014). The death rate was more than four times higher after a diagnosis of AD in people aged 75–84 and nearly three times higher in those aged 85 and older. More than one-third of total deaths in those age groups were attributable to AD with the average time from diagnosis to death about four years. After death, AD was confirmed through autopsy for about 90 percent of those who were clinically diagnosed. According to James et al. (2014), this translates into an estimated 503,400 deaths from AD in the US population over age 75 in 2010, which is over five times higher than the CDC's estimate.

AD is the only cause of death among the top ten that currently cannot be prevented, cured, or even slowed. It is also always fatal, thus no survivors (Sinclair 2016). Moreover, while deaths from other major causes have decreased, deaths from AD have increased in recent decades. For instance, between 2000 and 2015, deaths attributed to AD increased 123 percent, while those attributed to heart disease decreased 14 percent (Alzheimer's Association 2018). It should be noted that this increase reflects both changes in patterns of reporting deaths on death certificates and an actual increase in the number of deaths attributable to AD.

AD is more prevalent in certain demographic groups, thus complicating policy making. First, almost two-thirds are women. Mazure and Swendsen (2016) contend that sex differences in the brain have important implications for AD especially in the intermediate and advanced stages and that its consideration is essential for its understanding, treatment, and prevention. Not only does AD disproportionately affect women, in part because they live longer, but they also experience a faster progression of hippocampal atrophy than men (Ardekani et al. 2016). They also have different clinical presentations, with men exhibiting more aggressive behavior and comorbidity while women tending to have more affective symptoms and disabilities and longer survival times (Sinforiani et al. 2010). Interestingly, women who test positive for the ε4 allele of the apolipoprotein E gene are at greater risk of developing AD than are men with this allele (Xing et al. 2015). Testing for the effects of other genes by sex, instead of pooling data for both sexes, could facilitate efforts to develop different management strategies to better serve both men and women with AD (Mielke et al. 2014). In addition to differences in genetic or brain-based vulnerabilities and different neuropathologies, societal factors such as education and occupation levels and behavioral factors including diet, exercise, and tobacco and alcohol use that have been linked to AD also vary by sex.

Secondly, a review of numerous studies by an expert panel concluded that African-Americans are about twice, and Hispanics about one and one-half times, more likely to have AD than Caucasians (Yaffe et al. 2013). Variations in health, lifestyle, and socioeconomic risk factors across racial groups likely account for much of this variation in risk (Chin et al. 2011). Despite some evidence that the influence of genetic risk factors on AD may differ by race, genetic factors do not appear to account for the disparities among racial groups (Lines et al. 2014). Instead, health conditions such as cardiovascular disease and diabetes, that are associated with an increased risk for AD and are more prevalent in African-American and Hispanic populations, are believed to account for these differences (Clark et al. 2005). Whatever the ultimate reason, the disparity by race introduces sensitive political issues to AD policy.

THE GLOBAL IMPACT OF DEMENTIA

Although this book focuses on AD policy in the United States, it is important to view it as a global problem. Today, an estimated 47 million people live with AD worldwide, a number that is projected to rise sharply to more than 135 million by 2050. Although most attention has focused on AD in high-income countries (HICs), 58 percent live in low- and middle-income countries (LMICs) and that is expected to rise to 71 percent by 2050 (Prince et al. 2015). Moreover, increases in the next 20 years are predicted to be much steeper in LMICs than in HICs. Because population aging is occurring fastest in these countries, the bulk of the increase in AD will occur in those very regions where access to social protection, services, support, and care is severely limited. Given differential rates of population aging, numbers affected by dementia are expected to double in HICs but more than treble in LMICs by 2050.

Furthermore, more than half of the global increase will occur in G20 countries that are not members of the richest G7, including populous and rapidly aging middle-income countries Brazil, China, India, Indonesia, Mexico, and Turkey (Prince 2017). To date, a huge proportion of people with AD have not received a diagnosis and are thus unable to access care and treatment. Even when dementia is diagnosed, the care provided is often fragmented, uncoordinated, and unresponsive to the needs of people living with it and their caregivers. The World Health Organization (WHO) Global Action Plan (2017) calls for a public health approach with three core elements: raising awareness; ensuring universal coverage of basic health and social care; and focusing on promotion and prevention.

In population studies of LMICs, dementia is consistently the leading contributor to disability and dependence. Until recently, estimates of worldwide prevalence were hampered by an absence of evidence from LMICs, but new research with culturally valid methods suggests that age-specific prevalence and incidence is like that of HICs (Prince et al. 2015).

Although worldwide awareness of the need to invest in the development of treatment and care for dementia is growing, substantial challenges in achieving acceptable levels of coverage and access to care persist in LMICs. At present, people with AD receive a diagnosis late in the disease course, if at all; around half of the people affected are diagnosed in HICs, but less than 10 percent in LMICs.

Alzheimer's Disease International (ADI) contends that AD is one of the biggest global public health challenges facing our generation and that recent data suggests that the current burden and future impact have been underestimated, particularly for the Asia East and Sub-Saharan African regions (Wimo and Prince 2010). Among the chronic diseases, AD makes by far the largest single contribution to disability and needs for care among older people. It also has a huge economic impact. The total estimated worldwide cost is US$818 billion, or 1 percent of global GDP, and it will become a trillion-dollar disease by 2018 (ADI 2016). Costs will escalate proportionately with numbers affected and with increased demand for formal care services, particularly in LMICs. Public health and disease control measures, education, and other factors that enhance cognitive development can improve the brain health of those entering old age, but estimates suggest that such improvements in population health will do little to blunt the impending epidemic in LMICs. The best available evidence suggests that the age-specific prevalence of AD is unlikely to change significantly in coming decades, even if its incidence falls in response to improvements in public health, although this conclusion remains conditional given the limited data available on secular trends and the variation across models (Prince et al. 2016).

SUMMARY

AD and other dementias clearly present critical problems for the United States and globally. Unfortunately, despite over a half century of research, unlike other major diseases, we do not have a clear understanding of the causes of AD. This has led to numerous theories and purported solutions, though to date none has been successful in stemming AD. Additionally, AD affects many parties and requires labor-intensive personal care over a long period of decline. On the one hand are millions of patients and their family members who must often bear the burden of care for many years and health funders that must pay the mounting costs of AD. On the other hand, many sectors have high economic stakes in AD, from the politically powerful pharmaceutical and rapidly growing memory care industries, to the AD research community, to all the periphery commercial interests. The competing interests and demands of these many parties heighten the political tensions and raise an array of policy concerns. Chapter 2 describes the political context and discusses the exigent policy issues that AD raises for all governments.

REFERENCES

Abou-Saleh, M.T., C. Katona and A. Kumar (2011) *Principles and Practice of Geriatric Psychiatry*, 3rd ed. New York: John Wiley & Sons.

Alonso Vilatela, M.E., M. Lopez-Lopez and P. Yescas-Gomez (2012) "Genetics of Alzheimer's Disease." *Archives of Medical Research* 43: e622–e631.

Alzheimer's Association (2016) Tests for Alzheimer's Disease and Dementia. http://www.alz.org/alzheimers_disease_steps_to_diagnosis.asp.

Alzheimer's Association (2017) "Beta-amyloid and the amyloid hypothesis." https://www.alz.org/documents/national/topicsheet_betaamyloid.pdf.

Alzheimer's Association (2018) "Alzheimer's disease facts and figures." *Alzheimer's and Dementia* 14 (3): 367–429.

Ardekani, B.A., A. Convit and A.H. Bachman (2016) "Analysis of the MIRIAS data shows sex differences in hippocampal atrophy progression." *Journal of Alzheimer's Disease* 50: 3.

Bartus, R.T., R.L. Dean III, B. Beer and A.S. Lippa (1982) "The cholinergic hypothesis of geriatric memory dysfunction." *Science* 217: 408–14.

Baum, M.L. (2016) "Patient requests for off-label bioprediction of dementia." *Clinical Neuroethics* 25 (4): 686–90. https://doi.org/10.1017/S0963180116000402.

BCBS (2016) "Corporate medical policy: Genetic testing for Alzheimer's disease." https://www.bcbsnc.com/assets/services/public/pdfs/medicalpolicy/genetic_testing_for_alzheimers_disease.pdf.

Bernier, P.J., C. Gourdeau, P-H. Carmichael, J-P. Beauchemin et al. (2017) "Validation and diagnostic accuracy of predictive curves for age-associated longitudinal cognitive decline in older adults." *Canadian Medical Association Journal* 189: E1472–E1480.

Bowler, J.V. and V. Hachinski, eds. (2003) *Vascular Cognitive Impairment: Preventable Dementia*. Oxford: Oxford University Press.

Brier, M.R., B. Gordon, K. Friedrichsen, J. McCarthy et al. (2016) "Tau and Ab imaging, CSF measures, and cognition in Alzheimer's disease." *Science Translational Medicine* 3 (338): 338ra66.

Chin, A.L., S. Negash and R. Hamilton (2011) "Diversity and disparity in dementia: The impact of ethnoracial differences in Alzheimer disease." *Alzheimer Disease and Associated Disorders* 25 (3): 187–95.

Clarfield, A.M. (2003) "The decreasing prevalence of reversible dementias: An up-dated meta-analysis." *Archives of Internal Medicine* 163 (18): 2219–29

Clark, P.C., N.G. Kutner, F.C. Goldstein, S. Peterson-Hazen et al. (2005) "Impediments to timely diagnosis of Alzheimer's disease in African Americans." *Journal of the American Geriatrics Society* 53 (11): 2012–17

Francis, P.T., A.M. Palmer, M. Snape and G.K. Wilcock (1999) "The cholinergic hypothesis of Alzheimer's disease: A review of progress." *Journal of Neurology, Neurosurgery, and Psychiatry* 66: 137–47.

Frisoni, G.B., M. Boccardi, F. Barkhof, K. Blennow et al. (2017) "Strategic roadmap for an early diagnosis of Alzheimer's disease based on biomarkers." *The Lancet* 16 (8): 661–76.

Fukui, T. (2016) "Disentangling dementia from neuropsychological perspectives." *Japanese Journal of Neuropsychology* 32 (3): 229–38.

Genova, L. (2008) "Busting the myth of Alzheimer's." http://lisagenova.com/busting-the-myth-of-alzheimers-2/.

Hayden, E.C. (2008) "Alzheimer's tests under fire." *Nature* 455: 30.

Hodgson, L.J. (2011) "Strategizing about Alzheimer's." *The Gerontologist* 51 (6): 876–80.

Howard, R. (2005) "Vascular cognitive impairment: Preventable dementia." *American Journal of Psychiatry* 162 (1): 199–200.

Hurd, M.D., P. Martorell, A. Delavande, K.J. Mullen and K.M. Langa (2013) "Monetary costs of dementia in the United States." *New England Journal of Medicine* 368 (14): 1326–34.

Innes, A. (2009) *Dementia Studies: A Social Science Perspective.* London: Sage Publications.

James, B.D., S.E. Leurgans, L.E. Hebert, P.A. Scherr et al. (2014) "Contribution of Alzheimer's disease to mortality in the United States." *Neurology* 82 (12): 1045–50.

Jaret, P. (2014) "A test for Alzheimer's disease raises thorny ethical issues." *AARP Bulletin* (May). http://www.aarp.org/health/brain-health/info-2014/alzheimers-disease-blood-test.html?intcmp=AE-HEA-RELBOX.

Knapton, S. (2014) "Alzheimer's disease could be prevented after new blood test breakthrough." http://www.telegraph.co.uk/news/science/science-news/10951689/Alzheimers-disease-could-be-prevented-after-new-blood-test-breakthrough.html.

Kosik, K.S. and E. Clegg (2010) *The Alzheimer's Solution: How Today's Care is Failing Millions and How We Can Do Better.* Amherst, NY: Prometheus Books.

Lab Tests Online (2014) "Blood test shows very preliminary results in predicting Alzheimer disease." https://labtestsonline.org/news/140326alzheimer/.

Lerner, A.J. (2013) "Amyloid imaging: The court of public opinion." *Neurology* 81: 1108–09.

Lin, J.S., E. O'Connor, R. Rossom, L.A. Perdue et al. (2013) "Screening for cognitive impairment in older adults: An evidence update for the U.S. Preventive Services Task Force." Evidence Report No. 107. AHRQ Publication No. 14-05198-EF-1. Rockville, MD: Agency for Healthcare Research and Quality.

Lines, L.M., N.A. Sherif and J.M. Wiener (2014) *Racial and Ethnic Disparities among Individuals with Alzheimer's Disease in the United States: A Literature Review.* Research Triangle Park, NC: RTI Press.

Livingston, G., A. Sommerlad, V. Orgeta, S.G. Costafreda et al. (2017) "Dementia prevention, intervention, and care." *The Lancet*. https://doi.org/10.1016/S0140-6736(17)31363-6.

Loy, C.T., P.R. Schofield, A.M. Turner and J.B. Kwok (2014) "Genetics of dementia." *The Lancet* 383 (9919): 828–40.

Luan, K., J.L. Rosales and K.Y. Lee (2013) "Viewpoint: Crosstalks between neurofibrillary tangles and amyloidplaque formation." *Ageing Research Review* 12: 174–181.

Mazure, C.M. and J. Swendsen (2016) "Sex differences in Alzheimer's disease and other dementias." *Lancet Neurology* 15 (5): 451–52.

Mielke, M.M., P. Vemuri and W.A. Rocca (2014) "Clinical epidemiology of Alzheimer's disease: Assessing sex and gender differences." *Clinical Epidemiology* 6: 37–48.

Nakamura, A., N. Kaneko, V.L. Villemagne, T. Kato et al. (2018) "High performance plasma amyloid-β biomarkers for Alzheimer's disease." *Nature* 554: 249–54.

National Academies of Sciences, Engineering, and Medicine (NASEM) (2017) *Preventing Cognitive Decline and Dementia: A Way Forward*. Washington, DC: The National Academies Press.

PharmaFocus (2013) "Biomarkers in Alzheimer's disease." http://www.insightpharmareports.com/Affiliated-Reports/Global-Data/PharmaFocus--Biomarkers-in-Alzheimer-s-Disease/–.

Porteri, C., E. Albanese, C. Scerri, M.C. Carrillo et al. (2017) "The biomarker-based diagnosis of Alzheimer's disease: Ethical and societal issues." *Neurobiology of Aging* 52: 132–40.

Power, G.A. (2010) *Dementia Beyond Drugs: Changing the Culture of Care*. Baltimore, MD: Health Professions Press, Inc.

Prince, M.J. (2017) "Progress on dementia—Leaving no one behind." *The Lancet*. https://doi.org/10.1016/S0140-6736(17)31757-9.

Prince, M.J., A. Wimo, M. Guerchet, G.C. Ali et al. (2015) *World Alzheimer Report 2015: The Global Impact of Dementia: An Analysis of Prevalence, Incidence, Cost and Trends*. London: Alzheimer's Disease International.

Prince, M.J., G.C. Ali, M. Guerchet, A.M. Prina et al. (2016) "Recent global trends in the prevalence and incidence of dementia, and survival with dementia." *Alzheimer's Research and Therapy* 8: 23. https://doi.org/10.1186/s13195-016-0188-8.

Sabat, S.R. (2018) *Alzheimer's Disease and Dementia: What Everyone Needs to Know*. Oxford: Oxford University Press.

Sachdev, P.S., D. Blacker, D.G. Blazer, M. Ganguli et al. (2014) "Classifying neurocognitive disorders: The DSM-5 approach." *Nature Reviews Neurology* 10: 634–42.

Sinclair, N. (2016) "The financial and emotional toll of America's Alzheimer's problem." http://finance.yahoo.com/news/alzheimers-most-expensive-disease-

caregivers-cost-190758660.html;_ylt=A0LEV12541VYQZoAsQFXNyoA;_
ylu=X3oDMTEyaTkzYXJyBGNvbG8DYmYxBHBvcwMxBHZ0aWQDQjMy
MTlfMQRzZWMDc3I-.

Sinforiani, E., A. Citterio, C. Zucchella, G. Bono et al. (2010) "Impact of gender differences on the outcome of Alzheimer's disease." *Dementia* 30: 147–54.

Stites, S.D, J. Karlawish, K. Harkins, J.D. Rubright and D. Wolk (2017) "Awareness of mild cognitive impairment and mild Alzheimer's disease dementia diagnoses associated with lower self-ratings of quality of life in older adults." *The Journals of Gerontology, Series B: Psychological Sciences and Social Science.* https://doi.org/10.1093/geronb/gbx100.

Villemagne, V.L., W.E. Klunk, C.A. Mathis, C.C. Rowe et al. (2012) "Aβ Imaging: Feasible, pertinent, and vital to progress in Alzheimer's disease." *European Journal of Nuclear Medicine and Molecular Imaging* 39: 209–19.

Ward A, S. Tardiff, C. Dye and H.M. Arrighi (2013) "Rate of conversion from prodromal Alzheimer's disease to Alzheimer's dementia: A systematic review of the literature." *Dementia and Geriatrics Cognitive Disorders Extra* 3: 320–32.

Weuve, J., L.E. Hebert, P.A. Scherr and D.A. Evans (2014) "Deaths in the United States among persons with Alzheimer's disease, 2010–2050." *Alzheimer's and Dementia* 10: e40–e46.

Whitehouse, P.J. (2014) "The end of Alzheimer's disease—From biochemical pharmacology to ecopsychosociology: A personal perspective." *Biochemical Pharmacology* 88 (4): 677–81.

Whitehouse, P.J. and D. George (2008) *The Myth of Alzheimer's.* New York: St. Martin's Press.

Wimo, A. and M. Prince (2010) *World Alzheimer Report 2010: The Global Economic Impact of Dementia.* London: Alzheimer's Disease International.

Winblad, B., P. Amouyel, S. Andrieu, C. Ballard et al. (2016) "Defeating Alzheimer's disease and other dementias: A priority for European science and society." *Lancet Neurology* 15: 455–532.

WHO (2017) Draft global action plan on the public health response to dementia. Report by the Director-General. April 3. http://apps.who.int/gb/ebwha/pdf_files/WHA70/A70_28-en.pdf?ua=1 (Accessed June 26, 2017).

Wu, T-Y., C-P. Chen and T-R. Jinn (2011) "Traditional Chinese medicines and Alzheimer's disease." *Taiwanese Journal of Obstetrics & Gynecology* 50: e131–e135.

Xing, Y., Y. Tang and J. Jia (2015) "Sex differences in neuropsychiatric symptoms of Alzheimer's disease: The modifying effect of apolipoprotein E ε4 status." *Behavioural Neurology.* Published online October 11. https://doi.org/10.1155/2015/275256.

Yaffe, K., C. Falvey, T.B. Harris, A. Newman et al. (2013) "Effect of socioeconomic disparities on incidence of dementia among biracial older adults: Prospective study." *British Medical Journal* 347: f7051.

Zick, C.D., C.J. Mathews, J.S. Roberts, R. Cook-Deegan et al. (2005) "Genetic testing for Alzheimer's disease and its impact on insurance purchasing behavior." *Health Affairs* 24 (2): 483–90.

CHAPTER 2

Public Policy Context: Funding and Policy Initiatives

Abstract This chapter outlines the policy making process and the policy context of Alzheimer's disease (AD) and summarizes the broad range of issues surrounding it. It examines why AD promises to be a policy challenge well into the future as its prevalence and economic costs escalate. It details the economic and social costs of AD and illustrates how they threaten to bankrupt health care systems unless we develop adequate anticipatory policies to deal with the issues they raise. The chapter also examines the research funding for AD compared to other diseases and summarizes recent policy initiatives and commission and association reports to deal with the challenges it raises.

Keywords Research funding • Economic and social costs of AD • Health care • Policy making

Only the government has the legitimate authority to make decisions that are binding and carried out in the name of the entire population. Other organizations, such as medical associations and societies, make decisions that affect many individuals and might have a bearing on what the government ultimately does, but their policies are not binding on the population by force of law. Policy making in the United States is complicated by federalism where both the national and state, as well as local governments

© The Author(s) 2019
R. H. Blank, *Social & Public Policy of Alzheimer's Disease in the United States*, https://doi.org/10.1007/978-981-13-0656-3_2

have a role in framing AD policy, but even in unitary political systems like Britain, the multi-faceted and long duration of the disease means that policies can vary widely by locale.

The move of AD to the policy domain brings to the forefront political deliberations and divisions and places the resolution of issues in the milieu of interest group politics. Given the high economic, social, and personal stakes surrounding AD, conflict is unavoidable because each group has its own demands. AD must compete not only with non-health areas for its share of societal resources, but it is also in competition for public attention and political support with highly organized causes like breast cancer and AIDS, as well as other types of dementia. Also, within AD, there are constant battles among those with different theories of AD for their share of research funding and among research, public health, and care priorities, Given the complexities of AD, and the many parties with specific needs and demands, a united political front is unlikely. Moreover, because of the huge economic stakes involved, policy pressures surrounding AD are intense on numerous fronts, often rendering policy makers unable or unwilling to become involved. The Alzheimer's Association and other advocacy groups, therefore, face a constant struggle to maximize political and public support for AD.

The impact of AD goes well beyond the health care needs of the person affected. As AD inexorably progresses, the patient becomes increasingly dependent on others for basic daily care and routine tasks, a physically safe environment, and protection from exploitation or abuse. Addressing the diverse medical and social care needs of the growing population with AD requires the adoption of a multi-faceted policy framework and agenda that explicitly acknowledge the complex and unique needs of people with AD and the impacts it has on carers and society at large (Bynum 2014). Public policies related to social service providers; agencies that provide appropriate housing, financial, and legal services; and the judicial system must complement other policies focused on funding prevention and risk reduction, effective treatment development, and efficient health care delivery.

Policy Making for Alzheimer's Disease

Public policy can be categorized as one of three basic types: regulatory, distributive, or redistributive. Regulatory policies impose constraints or restrictions on the actions of groups or individuals: they provide rules of conduct with sanctions backed up by the authority of government.

Distributive policies are based on the notion of public goods, for example, goods and services that benefit all citizens, but which are unlikely to be attained by voluntary acts of individuals due to lack of sufficient resources. Public goods are defined by each society based on how broadly government responsibility is interpreted. Normally, distributive policies provide advantages or benefits to specific segments of society principally through the power of the purse. Considerable governmental activity revolves around the provision of public services, often without undue controversy until scarcity forces trade-offs to be made as to what groups get what goods. Redistributive policies, in contrast, are inherently controversial because they represent decisions by governments to alter the distribution of wealth or property among groups in society. The reallocation of resources can be deliberate such as highly progressive taxes or result from shifts in resources from the young to old or the healthy to unhealthy. It must be emphasized that all policies create winners and losers, although the mechanisms by which gains or losses ensue are often subtle.

Government involvement can occur at many points from the research and innovation stages, to placing a technology on the market, to its use by private individuals. It can be permissive, affirmative, regulatory, or prohibitive. The government always has the option of taking no action, thus permitting any activities by the private sector. It can also make affirmative policies that promote or encourage certain activities, for example, government funding of research or provision of services to facilitate more widespread use of a specific drug or procedure. The question of whether the government ought to be providing such encouragement, and if so how, is a subject of political debate. For instance, should public funds be used to pay for expensive, yet unproven, interventions for AD patients? Or, should private insurers be required to cover the potentially unlimited expense of treating an AD patient?

Although regulatory policy can be framed to apply solely to government-supported pursuits, usually it consists of rules governing activities across the public and private sectors. For instance, regulation can be used to ensure that standards of safety, efficacy, and liability are adhered to and that marketing of products is fair. Lastly, while far less common than regulation, prohibitive policies could be implemented that impose legal sanctions on a specific research activity or application as has been done with human cloning. Another form of prohibitive policy is to preclude public funding of specific areas of research and development (e.g., certain types of human fetal or embryo research) or specific procedures such as electro-shock therapy. It remains to be seen what, if any, areas of AD research are candidates for prohibition, but any such policy will reflect political motives or be a response to demands of interest groups, often on moral grounds.

Another critical policy issue involves questions of distributive justice, mainly involving the access to services, many of which are costly and are likely to become even more so with the proliferation of half-way treatments that might extend life but add little quality. While it is premature to speculate about the relative costs and benefits of yet undeveloped AD treatments, cumulatively their cost will be high. As such, these interventions also raise questions as to who gets high priority for use of these procedures, whether insurance companies must pay for what might be experimental treatments, and to what extent a government can or should regulate their use. If access is to be equitable and coverage universal, how will it be funded? Key AD policy areas include:

- *Research funding.* Funding policies are critical for research on the cause of AD, how to prevent it, how to detect it early and accurately, and how to slow, if not cure, it.
- *Health care.* Payment policy and regulatory functions in Medicare and Medicaid have direct implications for people living with AD who are the heaviest users of acute care.
- *Long-term care (LTC) services and support.* Payment policy for nursing homes and strategies to support community living are fundamental for AD patients, about 75 percent of whom will spend time in a nursing home at some stage.
- *Public health.* Addressing healthy lifestyle and risk factors and education are important for a public health approach to managing the growing burden of AD.
- *Housing and community services.* Critical for those who wish to remain in their homes are wide range of services including carer support, adult day care, and senior centers. These services are less costly than nursing home care, but less visible to federal policy makers because they primarily are organized on the local level.
- *Labor.* New policies needed to address the challenge of ensuring a competent and adequate workforce, especially for hands-on carers, such as personal care assistants, home health aides, and nursing assistants. At present about 80 percent of care is informal by family and friends, but this is changing.

- *Justice and law enforcement.* Relevant policies in the legal and law enforcement arena address issues that arise with substituted judgment and the need to provide protection from exploitation, abuse, and neglect. Abuse of AD patients by overworked and exhausted carers is a growing problem.

In summary, some of the major policy issues of AD that are covered in this book center on: funding and research priorities; regulating commercial interests; support for informal and formal caregivers; institutional versus home care; innovative treatment facilities; protection of AD patients; advance directives; treatment abatement; and physician-assisted death.

Although there has been increased political awareness of AD in the last decade and much has been done by practitioners, organizations, and the media to bring it out of the shadows, AD is just beginning to be a national priority (Ramnarace 2010). Given its increasing prevalence and mounting cost (see Box 2.1), this raises key questions as to how best to: secure an appropriate level of public research funding for AD; reduce its financial impact on families and society; regulate the far-reaching and lucrative AD industry; and ensure that governments, businesses, and the media effectively call attention to the threat it represents and work to implement workable and fair solutions. Recent policy initiatives represent preliminary steps in that direction.

Box 2.1 Social Justice and Utility

AD patients are generally viewed as burdensome, contributing little of positive value. There is widespread belief among clinicians that AD care is futile because available treatments do not alter the course and prognosis. There are also economic barriers to normalizing the experience of AD because good dementia care is expensive and implementing a nationwide policy of extensive AD care could bankrupt the health care system. A utilitarian viewpoint might argue against comprehensive AD care since directing resources to younger, more productive members of society maximizes average or overall utility. Accordingly, the principles of justice and beneficence that support comprehensive AD care might be at odds with a guiding utilitarian framework (Robbins and Bernat 2017).

Recent Alzheimer's Policy Activity

The National Alzheimer's Project Act (NAPA) passed unanimously in both Houses of Congress and was signed into law by President Obama in 2011 (Public Law 111-375). NAPA calls for a national strategic plan across federal agencies to address the escalating crisis of AD, and mandates the Secretary of the Department of Health and Human Services (DHHS) to establish the National Alzheimer's Project to:

1. create and maintain an integrated National Plan to overcome AD;
2. coordinate AD research and services across federal agencies;
3. accelerate the development of treatments to prevent, halt, or reverse its course;
4. improve early diagnosis and coordination of care and treatment;
5. decrease disparities in AD for ethnic and racial minority populations; and
6. coordinate with international bodies to fight AD globally.

The law also establishes the Advisory Council on Alzheimer's Research, Care, and Services (Advisory Council) and requires the Secretary of DHHS, in collaboration with the Advisory Council, to create and maintain a National Plan to Address Alzheimer's Disease. The first National Plan, released in May 2012, recognized AD as a major public health issue; provided a blueprint for coordinating efforts across the federal government; and outlined goals, strategies, and actions for eliminating the burden of the disease.

Supported by congressional appropriation beginning in fiscal year 2005, the CDC established the Alzheimer's-specific segment of the CDC's Healthy Aging Program, referred to as The Healthy Brain Initiative. The CDC joined with the AA and other groups, including the NIA at the National Institutes of Health (NIH), Administration on Aging, AARP, and other public and private sector organizations to launch the Healthy Brain Initiative and create a road map for a coordinated public health response across agencies and organizations. It offered a "synergistic" model based on several principles: a firm grounding in science; an emphasis on prevention; a community and population approach; and a commitment to eliminating disparities among groups. In July 2015, NIH released the first of what is to be an annual professional judgment budget for Congress estimating the costs of accomplishing the research goals of the National Plan.

In addition to enhanced activity at the federal level, plans to engage public health in assertive efforts to address AD and other dementias have been published in 43 states, the District of Columbia, and Puerto Rico, with another four states in the process of writing plans (Alzheimer's Association 2016b). Although they vary in focus and detail, most plans address the following topics:

- Increasing awareness of AD among the public
- Encouraging increased detection and diagnosis of AD
- Improving individual health care for those with AD
- Improving the quality of the health care system for those with AD
- Expanding the capacity of the health care system to meet the needs of those with AD
- Better equipping health care professionals to deal with individuals with AD
- Increasing the number of health care professionals needed to treat the growing aging and AD populations
- Improving services provided in the home and community to delay the need for institutionalized care
- Improving LTC, including assisted living, for those with AD
- Assisting unpaid AD caregivers
- Increasing research funding for AD
- Promoting activities that would maintain and improve brain health
- Improving data collection regarding AD and its public health burden
- Improving public safety and addressing safety-related needs of those with AD
- Addressing legal protections for, and legal issues of, individuals with AD
- Improving how government evaluates and adopts policies to help people with AD and their families

Despite their differences, these public policy statements all call for coordination of resources, better communication, awareness, and essential linkages. However, to achieve the ambitious outcomes envisioned in these plans and policies, resolute action is urgently required (Hoffman 2015).

THE ECONOMIC AND SOCIAL COSTS OF ALZHEIMER'S DISEASE

The most striking policy problems of AD relate to its cost. AD is the most expensive disease in the United States and is engulfing federal and state health care budgets and depleting the life savings of millions of victims and their families (Reid 2015). In 2017, the lifetime cost of care for a person with AD was estimated to be $329,360. The total national cost of caring for those with AD and other dementias for 2018 is estimated to be $277 billion (Alzheimer's Association 2018). Medicare and Medicaid cover nearly 70 percent of the total health and LTC costs, with out-of-pocket spending adding $46 billion. If no curative therapies emerge, by 2040 spending on dementia patients is estimated to be $1.2 to $1.6 trillion (Bynum 2014).

Since most persons with AD are over 65, Medicare bears most of the health care costs for their extensive use of hospital-based care. Similarly, because AD patients require extended LTC and frequently outlive their assets, Medicaid pays over 60 percent of nursing home care. The long duration of illness, often in a state of disability and dependence, contributes significantly to the impact of AD. Studies indicate that people aged 65 and older live an average of four to eight years after a diagnosis, yet some live up to 20 years. On average, a person with AD will spend 40 percent of their total time living in its most severe stage, much of this in a nursing facility. By age 80, nursing home admission is anticipated for 75 percent of people with AD compared with only 4 percent of those of that age without it. Two-thirds of those who die of AD do so in nursing homes, compared with 20 percent of people with cancer and 28 percent of those dying from all other conditions (Alzheimer's Association 2018).

Because the costs of AD are driven chiefly by compensating for lost function instead of treatment or prevention, only 16 percent of AD costs are direct medical costs, whereas 41.7 percent are informal-care costs and 42.3 percent social-care costs. In contrast, for diabetes the direct costs amount to over 80 percent of the overall economic burden of the disease, in part a reflection of the availability of effective medical therapy to manage glucose control, prevent complications when possible, and treat complications when they occur (Winblad et al. 2016). The entire global market for pharmaceuticals and diagnostics for AD was estimated to be $10 billion in 2015, only a small fraction of the total costs of the disease (Mordor Intelligence 2016). This highlights not only the absence of effective therapy for AD, but also the large opportunity for new treatment and care options.

In addition to the economic costs of AD, its burden includes the intangible costs of reduced quality of life and mortality. The primary measure of disease burden in health-economic evaluations is disability-adjusted life years (DALYs), which is the sum of the number of years of life lost due to premature mortality and the number of years lived with disability, totaled across all those with the disease. Using this measure, AD rose from the 25th most burdensome disease in the United States in 1990 to the 12th in 2010. No other disease or condition increased as much. In terms of years of life lost, AD rose from 32nd to 9th, again the largest increase of any disease. In terms of years lived with disability, AD went from ranking 17th to 12th, a jump matched only by kidney disease. Based on these numbers, AD is responsible not only for the deaths of ever more Americans, but also contributes to proportionally more cases of poor health and disability.

Total per-person health care and LTC payments in 2015 from all sources for Medicare beneficiaries with AD were three times as great as payments for other Medicare beneficiaries in the same age groups ($49,126 per person for those with AD compared with $15,550 per person for those without it). Moreover, total per-person Medicaid payments for Medicare beneficiaries with AD were 19 times as great as Medicaid payments for other Medicare beneficiaries. Medicaid paid an average of $26,837 per person for Medicare beneficiaries with AD living in an LTC facility, compared with an average of $590 for older adults without the diagnosis living in the community and LTC facilities (Alzheimer's Association 2016a).

Medical care for elderly people with AD in the last five years of life costs far more than care for other major killers like cancer and heart disease (Kelley et al. 2015). AD costs, on average, more than $287,000 over those five years. That compares to about $175,000 for heart disease and $173,000 for cancer care. Since health insurance covers about the same amount, approximately $100,000, for each of these diseases, many AD families are left covering the difference themselves: on average over $61,000 out-of-pocket for AD care, far more than the $34,000 that for those without it. In their seminal study of dementia costs, Hurd et al. (2013) found that raising the probability of dementia from 0 to 100 percent leads to additional social costs of between $41,689 and $56,290 per person per year, depending on the imputation method used. Furthermore, as noted earlier, because AD lingers for many years, or decades in some cases, the cost, for both government insurance programs and families, is exceedingly high (Reid 2015).

Researchers also have evaluated the additional or incremental health care and caregiving costs of AD when comparing people with and without it who have the same coexisting medical conditions and demographic characteristics. One group found that the incremental health care and nursing home costs for those with AD was $32,781 in 2015 (Hurd et al. 2013). Another study found that the incremental lifetime cost of AD was 70 percent higher for women than men, due to their greater risk of developing AD and being more likely to be widowed and living in poverty (Yang and Levey 2015). Except for drugs, the average per-person payments for health care services (hospital, physician, and other medical providers, nursing home, skilled nursing facility, hospice, and home health care) were higher for those with AD than for other Medicare beneficiaries in the same age groups. The fact that only payments for prescription drugs were lower for those with AD might reflect the lack of effective pharmacologic treatments now available (Alzheimer's Association 2016a).

Importantly, none of these figures include the onerous costs borne by informal caregivers. AD affects entire families who are most likely providing direct care and/or financial support. These caregivers experience stress on many levels and are at enhanced risk for an array of chronic conditions, family strife, financial strain, and pressure at work as well as an array of behavioral health complications (see Chap. 4). In addition, an estimated 250,000 children and young adults between ages 8 and 18 help to care for someone with AD in the United States (Alzheimer's Association 2016a). Therefore, AD carries far-reaching implications for the entire community well beyond the patient and his or her caregivers.

AD patients have more hospital stays, skilled nursing facility stays, and home health care visits than other older people. There are 538 hospital stays per 1000 Medicare beneficiaries aged 65 and older with AD compared with 266 hospital stays per 1000 beneficiaries without it. Based on data from the Health and Retirement Study and Medicare, after controlling for demographic characteristics, clinical characteristics, and health risk factors, individuals with AD had a 1.66 times greater risk of having a preventable hospitalization than those without AD (Alzheimer's Association 2016a).

The process of acute care also is more complicated for people with AD, with significant cost implications (ADI 2016). The impact of AD on length of stay was validated in an analysis of Hospital Episode Statistics from the British National Health Service (NHS) (CHKS 2012). After adjusting for age, gender, and clinical status, mean lengths of stay were 27 percent longer for inpatients with AD (13.6 vs. 10.7 days). The authors of the report attempted to calculate the annual cost to the NHS, accounting for costs incurred from excess lengths of stay, excess readmissions, and the impact of excess falls. For 2010, the costs for excess lengths of stay were £117.3 million, those for excess readmissions £122.5 million, and those for excess falls £25 million, amounting to £264.8 million overall. They noted, however, that these figures almost certainly represent an underestimation of the incremental costs given the likely underdetection and underrecording of AD during hospital admissions (CHKS 2012).

Similarly, there are 283 skilled nursing facility stays per 1000 beneficiaries with AD compared with 73 stays per 1000 beneficiaries for those without it. Moreover, individuals newly diagnosed with AD have higher health care use and costs in the year prior to diagnosis and in the two years after diagnosis than others (Suehs et al. 2013). Medicare Advantage enrollees with a new diagnosis of AD had $2331 more in health care costs (medical and prescriptions) in the year prior to diagnosis, $9333 more in costs in the year following diagnosis, and $5761 more in costs in the second year following diagnosis. In another study of pre-diagnosis health care costs, Medicaid enrollees with AD had $5549 more in health care costs in the year prior to diagnosis, with $3321 due to additional outpatient medical care and $1442 in additional home care and adult day care services (Geldmacher et al. 2013).

Finally, because of its long duration, AD raises severe difficulties regarding LTC funding. Only 58 percent of older adults with AD live in the community, compared with 98 percent of other older adults. Additionally, many AD patients receive paid services at home or in adult day care centers, assisted living facilities, nursing homes, or a combination of these at different times during the long course of the disease. The average costs of these services are high (assisted living, $43,200 per year, and nursing home care, $80,300 to $91,250 per year). Forty-two percent of residents in assisted living facilities and 45 percent of residents in residential care facilities had AD in 2010. Of all Medicare beneficiaries residing in a nursing home, 64 percent have AD (Alzheimer's Association 2016a).

The financial burden is particularly severe for African-Americans, those with less education, and widows (Kelley et al. 2015). African-Americans have significantly higher costs of care than whites, primarily due to higher levels of inpatient care and greater severity of illness. These differences, in turn, could be attributable to later-stage diagnosis that leads to greater disability while receiving care, delays in accessing timely primary care, or a lack of care coordination of services across providers. Additional research is urgently needed to explain the reasons for this race disparity.

Despite their high use of hospital care, the chief determinant of health care costs for the AD is nursing home and informal-care costs, a burden largely borne by individuals and families, particularly among minority groups. Medicare policy must acknowledge the considerable financial risk currently faced by AD beneficiaries and examine reforms that might mitigate these risks. Unfortunately, many structural barriers now hamper effective partnerships between family caregivers and other providers of care. The current stress on individual autonomy and safeguarding the privacy of personal health information can limit family caregivers' access to information that is appropriate and beneficial when they are responsible for coordinating care or managing treatments. Furthermore, medical providers often are not compensated for time spent educating family caregivers about patients' medical conditions and treatments (Wolff et al. 2016). Because of its importance, Chap. 4 covers LTC policy in more detail.

Research Funding for Alzheimer's Disease

There has been an escalation in the federal commitment to AD research in recent years, reflecting intensified national interest. In 2011, Congress initiated the National Alzheimer's Project which mandated the National Plan to Address Alzheimer's Disease in 2012 that set a target date of 2025 to develop methods of prevention and effective treatment. NIH played a lead role by redirecting $50 million in funding in fiscal year (FY) 2012 and allocating $40 million in FY 2013 to promising avenues of AD research. Also, with the expectation that a significant portion of the funds would be aimed at AD research, federal appropriations to the NIH budget were increased $100 million in FY 2014 and $25 million in FY 2015. NIH also doubled the $100 million going to the BRAIN (Brain Research through Advancing Innovative Neurotechnologies) initiative. Thus, NIH spending on AD research increased by roughly 30 percent from FY 2011 through FY 2015. Moreover, in 2015, Congress passed the Consolidated Appropriations Act, 2016 (P.L. 114-113) that called for an additional $350 million toward AD research. Most recently, in March 2018 Congress voted to include a $414 million increase for AD and dementia research funding at the NIH in the FY2018 budget. When this increase is signed into law, AD and dementia research funding at the NIH will exceed $1 billion (Alzheimer's News 2018).

While these recent funding increases are encouraging, AD remains underfunded compared to other diseases. The NIH spends over $6 billion a year on cancer research, over $4 billion on heart disease research, and over $3 billion on HIV/AIDS research. Thus, cancer gets about six times more funding than AD, but only about three times as many people have cancer. For AD funding to be on a par with other diseases, $2 billion a year is necessary (Reid 2015).

Similarly, a recent British study found that dementia research gets many times less funding than cancer even though its cost to society is far greater. Approximately 2.3 million people in Britain have cancer compared with 800,000 people suffering from dementia, but for each person from suffering cancer there is £241 spent on research, compared with £118 for those with dementia (Luengo-Fernandez et al. 2015). In 2012, the combined research funding allocated by the government and charities to cancer, coronary heart disease, dementia, and stroke was £856 million, almost two-thirds of which (£544 million) was allocated to cancer, one-fifth (£166 million) to heart disease, and just 11 percent to dementia. Although a separate multi-million-pound fund was launched to help establish a large-scale, international scheme to discover new drugs and deliver a cure by 2025, dementia remains underfunded when compared with the burden of disease. Some suggest the disparity may be driven by ageism and the belief that diseases like AD are an inevitable part of getting older (Knapton 2015).

With sufficient funding for AD research, there are many promising approaches that might pay off. First, it has been long known that people born with Down syndrome have a heightened propensity to develop the cranial plaques and tangles that characterize AD, but many Down patients never develop dementia. If we could understand why they avoid AD, we might be able to discover how to prevent AD among all people as they age. Another area of research that is worthy of more attention involves rheumatoid arthritis (RA) because people suffering from RA do not appear to develop AD as the same rate as those without it. Finding the cause for this connection might be another avenue to prevention. Although the original assumption was that the nonsteroidal anti-inflammatory drugs (NSAIDs) taken for arthritis pain warded off AD, extensive studies of NSAIDs all failed (Alzheimer's Association 2018). The fact remains, though, that we are far away from finding either sufficient prevention or cure for this complicated disease. Finding a solution is almost certainly going to require significant sums of federal research funding. Getting that additional funding, in turn, is going to require greater efforts to make AD one of the diseases that enjoy political favor, and, thus, the support of politicians (Hoffman 2015).

As noted earlier, another priority that is made in allocating funding for any disease, including AD, is what proportions go to medical research, care of existing patients, and health promotion and prevention programs. Although this is an issue with any disease, according to Whitehouse and George, the myth of AD is "causing us to waste massive resources in unwise quests for magic bullets to 'fix' brain aging—putting cure before care and intervention and trying to achieve dominance over a domain that will continue to resist our control" (2008: 14). Thus, Whitehouse (2014) and other critics of the conventional premise that we can cure AD through more investment of public and private funding consider this a poor use of resources and argue that we must reverse current funding priorities for the treatment of AD. Prevention and care should be viewed as more important than cure, because even if effective drugs are developed, they might improve mortality by keeping people out of nursing homes longer, but are unlikely to diminish the number of older people with cognitive impairment in the long term. Current drugs do not, and potential future drugs might not, improve quality of life and might even cause individuals to live longer with AD.

Accordingly, although biotechnology still deserves a reasonable investment of societal resources, it would be more productive to spend our resources on prevention doing things to protect our brains from cognitive loss such as physical exercise, clean drinking water devoid of toxins like lead and mercury that damage brain tissue, eating healthy, and building communities that can help AD families. Evidence presented in Chap. 4 suggests that psychosocial interventions, like educational and arts programs, and supportive information technology may be at least as important as the search for a cure and that providing home-like community-based programs should be more of a funding priority (Sabat 2008). According to Whitehouse (2014), however, the huge investment in developing drugs to prevent the formation of the allegedly toxic beta-amyloid plaque fragment has dominated the field for the past decade, monopolizing funding and blocking research into other areas of biological and psychosocial research including caregiving and prevention.

GLOBAL RESEARCH POLICY INITIATIVES

The Alzheimer's Association International Research Grant Program, through private sector philanthropic support, has invested over $405 million in AD grant proposals and is the highest-impact non-profit funder of AD research in the world, ranking behind only the Chinese and US governments (Alzheimer's News 2018). At the WHO-hosted Ministerial Conference on Global Action Against Dementia in Geneva in March 2015, the British Government announced that over US$100 million will be invested in a new global Dementia Discovery Fund (WHO 2015). Major pharmaceutical companies have committed in principle to investing in promising research efforts for dementia, along with the non-governmental organization Alzheimer's Research UK and the Government. At the Conference, 80 countries joined experts from the research, clinical, and advocacy communities to discuss how they could move to combat dementia at the global level. WHO committed to leading and coordinating efforts and pledged to establish a Global Dementia Observatory (GDO). There was a consensus on the need for coordinated efforts to track evolution of the disease burden, create policies to address the impact of dementia, and conduct research for treatment and improved, cost-effective care.

The GDO is a web-based data and knowledge exchange platform of key dementia information that is currently being developed by WHO. Its primary objectives are to collect and disseminate key dementia data from member states to support evidence-based service planning and strengthening of policies as well as health and social care systems and to provide access to the collated information at national, regional, and global levels supplemented by statistics from other available sources such as WHO's Global Health Observatory that is a gateway to health-related statistics for more than 1000 indicators for its 194 Member States organized to monitor progress toward the Sustainable Development Goals (WHO 2017). The GDO also makes available global and regional dementia reports and country-specific information sheets summarizing a country's system capacity to support people affected by dementia. In addition, the GDO provides the monitoring mechanism to track the implementation and progress of the global action plan on the public health response to dementia.

SUMMARY

The state of AD policy continues to be in flux. Although it has not yet received the attention of diseases like cancer, heart disease, and AIDS, it is changing as the costs escalate. The remaining chapters will examine the range of policy dimensions as they relate to the regulation of commercial interests, LTC, health promotion and prevention, and decision making at the end of life. Each of these areas raises not only generic health policy issues such as funding and provision of services, but also issues unique to AD due to the nature of a disease that results in cognitive decline and incapacity for decision making. Chapter 3 turns attention to the commercial aspects and big business surrounding AD. It demonstrates that the public fear of AD heightens the likelihood of exploitation of vulnerable people looking for a fix to dementia.

REFERENCES

Alzheimer's Association (2016a) "Alzheimer's disease facts and figures." *Alzheimer's and Dementia* 12 (4). https://www.alz.org/documents_custom/2016-facts-and-figures.pdf.

Alzheimer's Association (2016b) Alzheimer's Disease State Plans. http://act.alz.org/site/PageNavigator/state_plans.html.

Alzheimer's Association (2018) "Alzheimer's disease facts and figures." *Alzheimer's and Dementia* 14 (3): 367–429.

Alzheimer's Disease International (2016) *World Alzheimer Report 2016. Improving Healthcare for People Living with Dementia; Coverage, Quality and Costs Now and in the Future.* London: Alzheimer's Disease International.

Alzheimer's News (2018) "Congress prioritizes Alzheimer's and dementia research funding in 2018 budget." https://alz.org/news_and_events_105707.asp?WT.mc_id=enews2018_03_21&utm_source=enews-aff-38&utm_medium0=email&utm_campaign=enews-2018-03-21.

Bynum, J.P.W. (2014) "The long reach of Alzheimer's disease: Patients, practice, and policy." *Health Affairs* 33 (4): 534–40.

CHKS (2012) "An economic analysis of the excess costs for acute care for patients with dementia." CHKS, 2012. http://www.chks.co.uk/userfiles/files/Dementia_an_economic_analysis.pdf

Geldmacher D.S., N.Y. Kirson, H.G. Birnbaum, S. Eapen et al. (2013) "Prediagnosis excess acute care costs in Alzheimer's patients among a U.S. Medicaid population." *Applied Health Economics and Health Policy* 11 (4): 407–13.

Hoffman, D. (2015) "Looking at the future of Alzheimer's disease policy." *Health Affairs Health Policy Lab.* http://healthaffairs.org/blog/2015/07/14/looking-at-the-future-of-alzheimers-disease-policy/.

Hurd, M.D., P. Martorell, A. Delavande, K.J. Mullen and K.M. Langa (2013) "Monetary costs of dementia in the United States." *New England Journal of Medicine* 368 (14): 1326–34.

Kelley, A.S., K. McGarry, R. Gorges and J.S. Skinner (2015) "The burden of health care costs in the last 5 years of life." *Annals of Internal Medicine* 163 (10): 729–36.

Knapton, S. (2015) "Dementia research gets 13 times less funding than cancer, figures show." http://www.telegraph.co.uk/news/health/news/11532982/Dementia-research-gets-13-times-less-funding-than-cancer-figures-show.html.

Luengo-Fernandez, R., J. Leal and A. Gray (2015) "UK research spend in 2008 and 2012: Comparing stroke, cancer, coronary heart disease and dementia." *BMJ Open 2015*; 5: e006648. https://doi.org/10.1136/bmjopen-2014-006648.

Mordor Intelligence (2016) "Global Alzheimer's diagnosis and drugs market—Growth, trends and forecast (2016–2021)." http://www.mordorintelligence.com/industry-reports/alzheimers-diagnosisand-drugs-market.

Ramnarace, C. (2010) "The high costs of caring for Alzheimer's patients." http://www.aarp.org/relationships/caregiving/info-10-2010/the_high_costs_of_caring_for_alzheimers_patients.html.

Reid, T.R. (2015) "Where's the war on Alzheimer's?" *AARP Bulletin* (Jan/Feb). http://www.aarp.org/health/brain-health/info-2015/alzheimers-research.html.

Robbins, N.M. and J.L. Bernat (2017) "Should dementia be accepted as a disability to help restore hope during cognitive decline?" *AMA Journal of Ethics* 19 (7): 649–55.

Sabat, S.R. (2008) "A bio-psycho-social approach to dementia." In M. Downs and B. Bowers, eds., *Excellence in Dementia Care: Research into Practice.* Maidenhead: Open University Press.

Suehs, B.T., C.D. Davis, J. Alvir, D. van Amerongen et al. (2013) "The clinical and economic burden of newly diagnosed Alzheimer's disease in a medicare advantage population." *American Journal of Alzheimer's Disease and Other Dementias* 28 (4): 384–92.

Whitehouse, P.J. (2014) "The end of Alzheimer's disease—From biochemical pharmacology to ecopsychosociology: A personal perspective." *Biochemical Pharmacology* 88 (4): 677–81.

Whitehouse, P.J. and D. George (2008) *The Myth of Alzheimer's.* New York: St. Martin's Press.

Winblad, B., P. Amouyel, S. Andrieu, C. Ballard et al. (2016) "Defeating Alzheimer's disease and other dementias: A priority for European science and society." *Lancet Neurology* 15: 455–532.

Wolff, J. L., J. Feder and R. Schulz (2016) "Supporting family caregivers of older Americans." *New England Journal of Medicine* 375 (26): 2513–15.

WHO (2015) "Governments commit to advancements in dementia research and care." http://www.who.int/mediacentre/news/releases/2015/action-on-dementia/en/.

WHO (2017) "The global dementia observatory." http://www.who.int/mental_health/neurology/dementia/GDO/en/.

Yang, Z. and A. Levey (2015) "Gender differences: A lifetime analysis of the economic burden of Alzheimer's disease." *Women's Health Issues* 25 (5): 436–40.

CHAPTER 3

The Alzheimer's Marketplace

Abstract This chapter examines the commercial aspects and big business surrounding Alzheimer's disease (AD). It argues that the strong public fear of AD, heightened by often dramatic media coverage, heightens the likelihood of exploitation of vulnerable people looking for a fix to declining cognition. After examining the wide range of products being marketed and discussing the scientific evidence of medical and other treatment approaches, it argues for greater regulation particularly over direct-to-consumer marketing of purported remedies and even cures for dementia.

Keywords Exploitation • Regulation of dementia treatments • Big business surrounding AD

Although the burden of AD on health and social systems and on families that provide care for loved ones who suffer from it will continue to mount in the coming decades, at the same time many people are making their careers or huge profits from it. These include a flourishing AD research community, a huge pharmaceutical industry stake, and a burgeoning memory care industry. AD is a multi-billion-dollar industry and its label is driven in part by drug companies and researchers who use it to maximize research support of the disorder and sustain the clinical empire built around it (Whitehouse and George 2008). While regulatory frameworks

© The Author(s) 2019   45
R. H. Blank, *Social & Public Policy of Alzheimer's Disease in the United States*, https://doi.org/10.1007/978-981-13-0656-3_3

of various forms exist in these areas, they often are insufficient to stop less reputable interests from exploiting the situation for a profit.

THE FEAR OF ALZHEIMER'S DISEASE

While many Americans worry about staying physically healthy as they contemplate old age, losing their mental faculty is their biggest fear. For instance the Research!America Health Poll found that declining health is the number-one concern (37 percent), followed by financial worries (23 percent) and dependence on others (6 percent) (Research!America 2006). Asked their greatest fear about growing old, they mentioned losing mental capacity twice as often as declining physical ability (62 percent vs. 29 percent, respectively). The fear of forgetfulness has made deep inroads into the American psyche. This contagion of anxiety around memory loss is so strong that many older adults seek help for the kind of day-to-day forgetfulness that once was considered normal (Gullettemay 2011).

According to Whitehouse and George (2008) the medical story of AD generates fear, paranoia, angst, and stigmatization—its diagnosis can act as a death sentence of the mind. By trying to de-stigmatize cognitive decline with a disease label, we have made the isolation of the sufferers worse. Thus, instead of reducing anxieties about AD or the stigma surrounding it, heightened public awareness has increased fears among aging citizens. Hertogh (2005) agrees that many people, especially the elderly, are fearful of AD and view it as a humiliating affliction affecting self and personality. What they fear most are its effects on independence and competence. Others fear AD because they have seen a parent, a grandparent, or other relative experience the steady erosion of memory, cognition, and identity as the disease progressed. Now they worry whenever they misplace something or forget a name, and vow that they will do whatever they can to prevent or delay its onset (Draper et al. 2010).

A survey by the MetLife Foundation found that people over 55 dread getting AD more than any other disease except cancer. Moreover, over 60 percent were concerned that they may someday have to care for someone with AD. For Garrett (2013), the fear that cancer engendered is being replaced by "dementiaphobia." Even the words "Alzheimer's" and "dementia" arouse a degree of fear that heart attack, stroke, or COPD often do not. Although they all can kill, for many people the fear of losing "who one is" and becoming fully dependent on others is more horrifying. Moreover, it is not only older people who fear AD. A 2015 Harris Poll found that more than 75 percent of millennials, Generation Xers, and baby boomers worry about what will happen to their memory as they age (Kunkle 2015).

A British poll found that older people are more fearful of developing dementia than cancer (Telegraph 2014). Two-thirds of people over the age of 50 fear that they will develop the condition, while just one in ten said they were frightened about getting cancer and just under 4 percent about acquiring a heart condition. This apprehension is often magnified by advocacy groups, manufacturers of purported anti-aging products, and the news media which tend to embellish the dread of AD. It does not help that AD is often characterized negatively, described as "dying while alive," "a slow death," or a "fate worse than death." If, indeed, this has become the model that AD represents, and for which there is no foreseeable cure, it is not surprising that many people view a loss of cognitive self and subsequent loss of autonomy as a dismal fate (Gordon 2015) (Box 3.1).

Box 3.1 Fear and Stigma of Dementia
In January 2018, the Alzheimer Society of Canada released the results of a survey of 1500 Canadians and found that 46 percent would feel ashamed or embarrassed if they had dementia. Moreover, 58 percent believe that people with AD or another form of dementia are likely to be ignored or dismissed, 57 percent be taken advantage of, and 37 percent feared or met with distrust or suspicion. While 56 percent of Canadians are concerned about being affected by AD—of greatest concern is their fear of being a burden to others, losing their independence, and the inability to recognize family and friends—only 39 percent would offer support for family or friends who were open about their diagnosis, and 30 percent admit to using dementia-related jokes (http://alzheimer.ca/sites/default/files/2018-01/Awareness2018-en.pdf).

As Draper et al. (2010) note, however, the lived experience of AD can differ from the imagined experience. Although the debilitating impact of AD cannot be minimized, their literature review of the personal experiences of patients living with it found no solid support to the widespread view that AD is a "dreadful state of suffering." Overall, those with early and mid-stage AD have more positive appraisals of their lives than expected and can enjoy human interactions and mental and physical activity, even as the disease progresses (de Boer et al. 2007). Up to 67 percent of people with mild to moderate dementia report a good or very good quality of life (Draper et al. 2010). In other words, those suffering most might be those who see AD from the outside.

Sabat (2018) argues that the rhetoric surrounding the care of AD patients and that is endemic in current medical practice is part of a "deficit approach," which focuses overwhelmingly on problems and limitations. He challenges the detrimental stereotypes of AD sufferers that they are passive, vegetables, antisocial, or irrationally angry because they make it easier to mistreat and misinterpret them. Many persons with AD are hardly as disabled as they are socially expected to be. What he terms "learned helplessness" is a reaction to stereotyping and acts as a self-fulfilling prophecy, since their symptomatic behavior is largely a response to the stereotypes that others project onto them, along with self-stereotypes that they have learned and absorbed. Those diagnosed with AD can be passive and apathetic, but it is principally the result of the social isolation that they frequently experience (Sabat 2018).

Despite these more optimistic perspectives, the fear of AD is widespread and the threat of developing it does create a vulnerability to pursue aggressively marketed products and technologies that promise to prevent or cure it, even though none enjoy proven effectiveness. This summary of two respondents of a study by Kunkle (2015) elucidates the extent of this quest for protection from AD. "It's my nightmare: the loss of my mind; the inability to recognize people who are dear to me; the ability to think," said one 71-year-old man, whose mother had AD. He does everything he can to lower his risk, including working out, reading vociferously, doing crossword puzzles, eating almonds, and following the news about possible new treatments. Another interviewee eats blueberries every day, works out for strength and aerobics, does word puzzles, and is learning Spanish. Should she develop AD, she will move to a state that permits euthanasia so that she can die in peace and not be a burden because there is "nothing worse than this disease." Although there is nothing inherently harmful about these individuals' lifestyle choices, their lives have become, in effect, captured by a fear of AD.

COMMERCIALIZATION AND MARKETING OF ALZHEIMER'S PRODUCTS

The fear of AD has not been lost on an emergent industry that focuses on products that promise to improve cognition and, in many cases, avert AD or even cure it. A quick search of AD on the Internet finds countless sites to this end. AD is big business as illustrated by the thousands of items on Amazon.com alone. According to Conrad and Horwitz (2013), medicalization of cognitive issues is linked to the availability and profitability of treatment options, buoyed by a growing consumerist orientation to health and reinforced by enthusiastic media reporting. Moreover, the Internet enables consumers to access AD products without the need to visit a doctor, thus illustrating medicalization via the application of a medical solution to an everyday problem, often under a new diagnostic category. One example is the emergence of the recent disease and susceptibility category of mild cognitive impairment (MCI) which elucidates how blurry the boundaries are between what is normal and abnormal cognitive functioning and how they can shift quickly (Coveney et al. 2011).

Both the popular press and, especially, the Internet are predisposed to highly optimistic and oversimplified coverage of all biomedical technologies. In addition, health-oriented magazines and television shows extol the virtues of innovations and the quick fixes or breakthroughs these innovations might offer. By and large, then, media coverage solidifies public trust in the technological fix and stimulates its appetite for new, often expensive, high-technology procedures. For instance, Gilbert and Ovadia (2011) document many instances of hype and exaggerated coverage of deep brain stimulation (DBS) in both scientific journals and the popular press. Even Nature presented DBS findings in an overly optimistic article entitled "Brain electrodes can improve learning" that was quickly followed by enthusiastic coverage in television news and the press that headlined "Deep stimulation 'boosts memory' " (Gilbert and Ovadia 2011).

Direct-to-consumer advertising refers to a variety of marketing practices based on a combination of information and promotion strategies directed at consumers through media such as television (often late night), newspaper and magazine ads, and, of increasing consequence, the Internet. Direct-to-consumer advertising of drugs has been legal in the United States since 1985, but it accelerated in 1997 when the FDA eased up on a rule requiring companies to offer a detailed list of side effects in their infomercials. Since then, the pharmaceutical industry has poured billions into this form of promotion. Direct-to-consumer advertising in the United States has contributed to burgeoning drug marketing and sales in the past decades once companies were permitted to advertise. Although proponents argue this marketing introduces the public to innovations, empowers patients, and provides updated health information directly to potential users, critics argue that it is used to drive choice, rather than inform it, by persuading patients to ask their doctor to prescribe a specific drug, most likely an expensive one (Humphreys 2009). It is also blamed for encouraging so-called off-label uses of drugs, uses not approved by the FDA.

With drug companies on the defensive in the United States, they have actively attempted to push into markets where direct-to-consumer advertising is not yet permitted such as the European Union, mostly without success. The only other country in the world that allows direct-to-consumer drug ads is New Zealand. Palmour and Racine (2011) view such marketing of dietary supplements to maintain or enhance cognition as an unhealthy commerce of neuroscience.

The Internet and emails, often through fabricated "news" stories, have facilitated marketing of all sorts of products that claim to prevent, slow, and even reverse or cure AD that are targeted to anxious seniors. Below are a few excerpts from some of these sales pitches:

1. Discover the cooking oil that repairs memory. During this short video you will also discover how much of this oil you need to take each day to repair and boost memory, increase focus and concentration and **prevent and reverse Alzheimer's and dementia**. And do it in just 21 days.

2. In the October 2012 issue of *Natural Health Dossier*, we revealed the top three natural treatments that **can not only prevent Alzheimer's—but also reverse it**. Simple, natural ways to protect your brain and preserve your memory.

3. **Chewy Snack Shuts Down Alzheimer's Research?** The Alzheimer's-reversing power of THIS chewy snack *virtually* **shut down research at one of the biggest pharmaceutical companies**. Why? Because the memory-boosting power of this snack is so powerful, **medical experts are coining it "THE ALZHEIMER'S DISCOVERY" of the century**. *I thought this was impossible too…* Until I saw this chewy snack **reverse *even the most severe* cases** of Alzheimer's and dementia. So, if you are at all worried about your own memory, then you **MUST** stock up on this chewy superfood **IMMEDIATELY**.

4. This is a HUGE breakthrough. According to a team of 31 senior scientists at Oxford …Alzheimer's and dementia are caused by common viral infections. **Now the good news is that scientists have discovered a way to quickly destroy these Alzheimer's germs.** That's probably why many health experts are calling this the health breakthrough of the 21st century. People are using this natural "antibiotic" to kill their Alzheimer's infection in under a month… **And data is showing it works for all stages of Alzheimer's and dementia—no matter how severe.**

5. Quick and Natural Alzheimer's Cure Could Be Extinct by June 1st, 2017? Over 142 grocery stores affected in your area alone! Stay on this page to find out how to get your hands on this **DEMENTIA-ERASING** superfood before it runs out.

6. A journey that opened my eyes to the sick, predatory, and ultimately deadly practices of the pharmaceutical conglomerates that would eventually lead to the discovery of a completely natural, 100% effective way that could **reverse even the most severe cases of Alzheimer's… No matter whether one suffering was in the very late stages, at initial onset, or simply at risk of age related memory loss.** It's A Method That's Based on Breakthrough Research Conducted by A Team of Scientists at Yale University…It's already been proven to be effective…And all it takes is the destruction of a simple "evil agent" in your brain…that has now been pinpointed as the overwhelming cause of almost all memory-destroying diseases.

7. We're no longer talking about just slowing mental decline, **but actually STOPPING and REVERSING it. Bringing back FULL brain function**—memories, intelligence, quick thinking, even sense of humor…Can you imagine your loved one getting back to their old self…a few short months from now? Lost memories coming back…the brain fog vanishing…clear thinking returning…And here's the best news of all: The ICT protocol is something you can do on your own, at home.

8. **YES!** Send me my **FREE Alzheimer's & Memory Loss Prevention Package** and Bonus Report from renowned brain expert Dr. Gary Small. I will receive my Package for agreeing to try a subscription to **Mind Health Report** at the low rate of only $54.95 for a year (12 monthly issues)

9. ★ This 4 Course Meal Plan **Reverses Alzheimer's** ★

10. Dr. Oz suggests eating curry once or twice a week (or curcumin supplements) to help **prevent Alzheimer's disease.**

11. Pure Essence Cannabidiol (CBD) Oil is found to have benefits as a neuroprotectant, for example in limiting neurological damage following stroke and trauma, **or in the treatment of neurodegenerative diseases,** such as Alzheimer's and Parkinson's.

12. Could the type of shampoo you use cause Alzheimer's disease? Recently, the NIH studied the most popular shampoo brands and discovered that 4 brands contain a deadly chemical that causes your brain to "shut down" and eventually, develop Alzheimer's disease. When you click here now and watch this short presentation, you'll discover the **ONLY known cure for Alzheimer's disease.**

13. **By simply eating this sweet snack 30 minutes before bed, you can reverse Alzheimer's disease…**Think that's impossible? Then listen to this…Recently, one Harvard-recognized doctor revealed how this food helps dissolve deadly brain plaque while you sleep… **Results were so powerful, medical experts are calling it THE ANSWER to Alzheimer's.** If you ever worry that your memory is getting worse… or if a loved one is suffering with Alzheimer's or dementia… this 1 food could be a life-saver. P.S. This pre-bed "recipe" **is perfectly simple to make… but you have to know the right way to prepare it.** You'll get everything you need in this short video. Click here now to discover this Alzheimer's-reversing food…

14. New research reports that THIS everyday bathroom habit is now a leading cause of memory loss and Alzheimer's. So what is this everyday bathroom habit that's killing your brain cells, destroying your memory, and increasing your risk of Alzheimer's and dementia? Watch this video to find out—you will also discover a breakthrough technique that thousands have been using to boost their brain health, dramatically improve their memory, vision and **even reverse Alzheimer's and dementia permanently—and in as little as 14 days.**

15. Breaking News: Natural Alzheimer's cure which **kills disease in Just 21 days**—Click below to get this natural cure without expensive meds which can make you worse…

16. Unfortunately, most people just don't have enough magnesium ions available. In Dr. Dean's book *The Magnesium Miracle*, you will find help for many chronic diseases and conditions linked to inflammation. Take **Alzheimer's**, for example. Magnesium blocks the inflammation caused by deposits of calcium and other substances in brain cells. While magnesium is one of the safest nutrients you can take, you need to know what you're doing to optimize your magnesium levels for better health. That's why Dr. Dean's book is indispensable.

Moreover, in their quest for a wider market, the brain intervention industry has distorted the line between therapy and enhancement (Blank 2015). If it works for AD patients, it can enhance cognition of healthy people. Dr. Oz says: "It's the future of the brain," the World's 11th richest man says that since taking this IQ-boosting pill his creativity, problem-solving, and focus have increased significantly, and CNN Breaking News reports that this "clear-pill" is so effective, that the government is thinking about banning it. Interestingly, the name of this wonder supplement varies, Alpha ZXT and Geniux, among others. The ads even include "limited edition cover pages" of magazines such as National Geographic, Forbes, and Time extolling the pill that can turn you into "the quickest thinker on the planet!" According to their website, Geniux has been clinically proven to "sky-rocket concentration by 312 percent, improve creative thinking, boost energy, enhance memory recall and increase IQ scores by 77 percent." Similarly, Alleradd is marketed as a nutritional supplement available online to anyone with a valid credit card who states they are at least 18. Another widely marketed pill is Addium termed "Viagra for the brain" and "the most powerful brain enhancer in the world" by a group of television "doctors." Interestingly, in almost identical ads, the same compound is called Adderin, Geniux™ (medical name E-Huperzine), and Alpha ZDT!

These types of marketing have led to a call for greater regulation over direct-to-consumer advertising of brain intervention products (Hanrahan 2013). Certainly, there is a clear regulatory gap for neurotechnologies with non-therapeutic and non-diagnostic commercial purposes. As argued by Racine et al. (2007), the commercial development of neurotechnologies deserves greater regulatory attention because of the exceptional ethical questions they evoke. At the very least, consumer protection from false advertising and to guard against potential long-term safety problems are imperative in the growing commercialized cognitive-product environment.

CURRENT ALZHEIMER'S DRUGS

The drugs currently approved by the FDA for AD target biochemical abnormalities. Although they might temporarily improve symptoms or mask them in some patients, they do not modify the underlying neuropathology or its progression and none of them slows or stops the damage and destruction of neurons that cause AD symptoms and make it fatal (Yuan et al. 2015). Furthermore, their effectiveness varies from person to person. For example, three cholinesterase inhibitors—donepezil, rivastigmine, and galantamine—are in routine use, but none has shown neuroprotective potential in humans. The latest drug to treat the symptoms of AD at the moderate to severe stages approved in 2014 by the FDA is a combination of donepezil and memantine (Namzaric).

Between 2002 and 2012, 244 drugs for AD were tested in clinical trials but only one successfully completed the trials and received FDA approval (see Box 3.2). In 2017, Merck halted the late-stage trial of its highly touted drug verubecestat, after an independent study found that it had "virtually no chance" of working. This came just three months after Eli Lilly announced that it was ending the clinical trial of its AD drug solanezumab, after patients taking it demonstrated no signs of improvement compared to a placebo. This humanized monoclonal antibody was designed to increase the clearance from the brain of soluble $A\beta$ peptides. However, at a dose of 400 mg administered every four weeks in patients with mild AD, it did not significantly affect cognitive decline (Honig et al. 2018). Similarly, in February 2017, Lundbeck announced its 5-HT6 antagonist had failed two key trials, quashing any last hopes for that drug. Axovant, whose drug aims to treat the symptoms of AD, had phase-3 data coming out in late 2017, but some of its competitors pursuing the same target have had disappointing results. Although there have been many successful studies that have cured or reduced memory loss in transgenic lab animals, none have been replicated in humans (Cummings et al. 2017). Apparently, mice AD is easier to treat than the human variety.

Box 3.2 Continued Bad News
2018 started out as a disheartening year for research into drug treatments for AD. Negative results have been posted for phase III clinical trials of two 5-hydroxytryptamine-6 receptor (5-HT_6) antagonists for the symptomatic treatment of moderate dementia, as well

as for a trial of an amyloid β antibody as a disease-modifying treatment in mild dementia. Pfizer announced that it will end its neuroscience and related dementia investments in drug development, removing a major industry partner from the field. These developments follow a long period of negative drug trials in AD. Over the past decade, the failure rate has been nearly 100 percent, and the only registered medicines are the cholinesterase inhibitors and memantine, which at best generate modest symptomatic improvement in cognitive testing among some patients and for only a short time (Le Couteur et al. 2018).

Brain Games: Computer-Based Cognitive Training

The range of cognitive intervention includes not only pharmacological interventions, but also psychological interventions, such as learned tricks or mental strategies, as well as external technological and institutional structures that support cognition. There are three popular computer-based approaches to improving cognition: brain-training programs; working-memory training; and video-game training (Boot and Kramer 2014). Computer-based cognitive-training software, popularly known as brain games, are aggressively marketed, especially to aging adults. Products in this billion-dollar industry include Cogmed, Posit Science, and Lumosity, which alone has over 60 million members and advertises extensively even on NPR classical music stations. Although the premise is similar across these products, their emphasis varies.

The promotion of these products entices and reassures a worried public. Consumers are told that playing brain games will reduce cognitive slowing and forgetfulness and improve one's mind. It is customary for advertising to highlight the benefits in abstract terms and assure consumers that its claims and promises are based on scientific evidence often designed by neuroscientists at "top universities and research centres" (Ghoravshi 2014). In many instances, however, the cited studies embody something other than the program being advertised, assessing benefits with abstract laboratory tasks rather than everyday ones (Boot and Kramer 2014). There is evidence that brain training can produce improvement in practiced skills that might extend to improvement on other cognitive tasks. However, in commercial promotions, these small, narrow, and fleeting advances are often billed as general and lasting improvements of the brain (Max Planck Institute 2014). Moreover, cognitive activity takes many forms, and there is currently little evidence suggesting that any software package improves cognition, or that any brain-training product is better than other brain-engaging activities such as learning a new language or musical instrument, creative writing, or aerobic exercise (Boot and Kramer 2014).

The largest study of brain training was Brain Test Britain with over 11,000 participants aged 18–60 who were randomly assigned to receive reasoning training and general brain training like that of commercial brain-training games. Although the subjects demonstrated improved proficiency on the specific brain-training tasks, this did not translate to significant benefit in standardized cognitive assessments of executive function, attention or working memory (Owen et al. 2010). Longer-term benefits in reasoning, verbal learning, and activities of daily living (ADLs) were reported for the over-age 50 participants, but there was a substantial number of dropouts after 12 weeks (Corbett et al. 2015).

Concerns over the marketing claims by some of these companies led a group of 73 international psychologists, cognitive scientists, and neuroscientists to write an open letter accusing them of exploiting the anxiety of adults facing old age for financial gain by making exaggerated and misleading claims not based on sound scientific evidence (Max Planck Institute 2014). Moreover, the promise of a magic bullet detracts from the best evidence to date that cognitive health in old age reflects the long-term effects of healthy, active lifestyles. Thus, promoting computer games as a fix to deteriorating cognitive performance diverts attention and resources from legitimate prevention efforts. Perhaps the most pernicious claim is that brain games prevent or reverse AD (Redick et al. 2013).

Neurofeedback Training

Neurofeedback uses real-time displays of brain activity utilizing neuroimaging with a goal of enabling the person to regulate his or her brainwave activity through a process of operant conditioning (Sulzer et al. 2013). Connected to a computer, the person receives instantaneous auditory and visual feedback about brainwave activity. With repeated feedback training and practice, desirable brainwave patterns can usually be retrained in most people. In the clinical domain, neurofeedback has been used to treat patients with attention deficit/hyperactivity disorder (ADHD), epilepsy, and autism, but increasingly, it is being used in healthy individuals to enhance attention and memory. Already, there are many websites, as well as non-medical clinics, selling basic neuro-feedback devices and equipment designed to improve cognitive performance and other functions (Maslen et al. 2014).

Despite limited evidence, neurofeedback training is being promoted as a therapy to help with memory lapses and MCI. The training involves recording a person's brain waves while he or she watches a video. If these brain waves show that the person has become inattentive, the screen momentarily flickers or blurs, forcing the person to focus on it again. Presently, neurofeedback training, which costs about $100 per session, requires 30–40 sessions. In a small German study, Hohenfeld et al. (2017) found that healthy elderly and patients with prodromal AD showed improved visuospatial memory performance and performed better in a working-memory task after neurofeedback training. If supported by ongoing large-scale clinical studies assessing the potential benefits of neurofeedback training in MCI and AD, these findings suggest that cognitive decline might be offset using fMRI-based neurofeedback.

Physical Interventions in the Brain

The failure of current drugs to treat AD has also led to alternative or complementary therapeutic treatments. Non-pharmacological interventions including "non-invasive" brain stimulation techniques such as transcranial magnetic stimulation (TMS) and transcranial direct current stimulation (tDCS), often in combination with cognitive training, have gained media attention. TMS employs a coil to deliver brief magnetic pulses to the scalp, inducing electric currents in the targeted areas of the brain (Hsieh 2015). Compared to TMS, tDCS stimulators are typically inexpensive, battery-operated, and portable and have safety advantages, with no reported serious adverse effects (Mrakic-Sposta et al. 2016). Elder and Taylor (2014) evaluated the effects of TMS and tDCS on cognitive and neuropsychiatric symptoms in the major dementias and concluded that both have potential as interventions for the treatment of AD and MCI. Post-rTMS improvements in depression and cognition have been demonstrated in mild to moderate, but not severe, AD patients.

Proponents of these techniques argue that the application of cognitive rehabilitation at an early stage is crucial since some aspects of cognitive functions are preserved until later in AD (Cotelli et al. 2014). One study found that a single tDCS session can ameliorate memory deficits in AD patients (Ferrucci et al. 2008). Moreover, Boggio et al. (2009) demonstrated that repeated sessions of anodal tDCS applied bilaterally over the temporal area led to an increase in performance of visual recognition memory tasks in a group of AD patients. Marceglia et al. (2016), too, found that the abnormal pattern of EEG activity observed in AD during memory processing is partially reversed by applying anodal tDCS. As Meinzer et al. (2015) point out, the long pre-clinical phase of AD provides opportunities for potential disease-modifying interventions in prodromal stages. Although the possibility of tDCS as a full-fledged treatment for AD is not imminent, research demonstrates its potential use to help alleviate some of its major symptoms. Given its simplicity and the amount of research support for tDCS, it could become a generalized therapeutic tool, but as Drakos (2015) warns, we must beware the commercial exploitation of this technology because if used in the wrong way, it can be harmful.

Deep brain stimulation (DBS) is a surgical procedure in which electrodes are implanted into targeted areas providing a steady stream of electrical impulses to a part of the brain that regulates memory. Early research indicated that DBS, which is commonly used to treat the symptoms of chronic pain, major depression, and PD, could slow down or even halt cognitive decline in AD patients (Laxton et al. 2010). A recent study of 42 patients with mild AD found that over a 12-month period, those aged 65 and over who received DBS saw "a trend toward ... benefit on clinical outcomes" and a possible "slowing of cognitive decline," although younger patients did not benefit from the treatment and may have worsened (Novacic 2016).

During a five-hour surgery in 2015, Kathy Sanford became the first AD patient in the United States to have a DBS stimulator implanted in her brain as one of up to ten patients enrolled in a clinical study (Lozano et al. 2016). Using a three-dimensional brain mapping technique called standardized low-resolution brain electromagnetic tomography (sLORETA), Lozano's group found that stimulating the hypothalamus also produced increased brain activity in the hippocampus, a key component in the brain's memory circuitry. As AD progresses, not only does the hypothalamus atrophy, but electrical communication between neurons in the region also gradually becomes impaired. Regretfully, after one year there were no significant differences in cognition between the groups, although because AD tends to progress slowly, reversing or slowing the degeneration associated with condition may take more time to become noticeable. Laxton and Lozano (2013), however, warn that evidence for the use of DBS to treat AD is preliminary and limited, and that further investigation into its potential clinical effects is warranted.

Despite the uncertain efficacy of these interventions to date, according to one website, researchers have been studying the benefits of tDCS for years, and the results they have uncovered are "astounding." The Brain Stimulator proclaims it is the industry leader and sells a wide range of products including the $90 Full Featured Brain Stimulator and the $55 Brain Stimulator Travel Model. Among the "endorsements" noted are a TV doctor, an article in the New Yorker, and a PBS story. Another example of the marketing of tDCS comes from the Brain Stimulation Clinic that advertises that it is a safe, new, non-invasive procedure which improves attention, memory, and learning for healthy individuals and patients with disabilities. Moreover, it can be performed at the clinic in Atlanta or self-administered with training and supervision through the Home-Use Program.

STEM CELL THERAPY

The failure to develop new drugs for AD also intensified attention to stem cells in 2010 when researchers began clinical trials investigating their use for AD. Two phase-1 trials on moderate AD patients have been completed and, although they revealed no severe acute or long-term side effects, no significant clinical efficacy was observed. Several studies, which involve more sophisticated study designs using different injection routes and biomarkers such as amyloid PET, are planned for mild to moderate AD patients (Kang et al. 2016). Based on preliminary findings, the Alzheimer's Society supports a legislative environment that allows stem cell research to develop within a strict regulatory framework (Thraves 2015). Cote et al. (2017), however, argue that many of the stem cell transplants in neurologic diseases are unproven and have never been tested in prospective, controlled clinical trials. Such procedures are presented as therapy but remain experimental and unregulated and could put patients at risk. Moreover, some current stem cell interventions for neurologic diseases are ethically dubious because patients are not included in a clinical trial or they do not offer genuinely informed consent.

Despite limited evidence of efficacy, however, stem cell treatments for AD are being marketed. StemGenex Medical Group (2016) provides stem cell therapy to help patients who fail to respond to typical drug treatment, want to reduce their reliance on medication, or want to try stem cell therapy before starting drug treatment. Similarly, Stem Cell Therapy Plus advertises that it is "giving new hope" to AD patients.

> Anecdotal evidence shows that the usage of Stem Cell Therapy Plus retards the degenerative process associated with this disease and improves the efficiency of traditional drug treatments.... Unlike traditional Stem Cell Therapy which can only be applied via injection in the selective hospitals/clinics, Stem Cell Therapy Plus delivers stem cells through high-tech bioactive softgel capsules which can be delivered right to your home. All you need to do is to take 1–3 softgel capsules a day at the comfort of your own home (2016).

Likewise, the Harvard Stem Cell Institute (HSCI) uses induced pluripotent stem cell technology to direct patient stem cells to become brain cells both affected and not affected by AD. They argue that while none of the FDA-approved treatments on the market for AD confront the underlying cause of the disease, by using stem cells HSCI scientists can reveal potential targets for therapeutic intervention. This is done by studying the differences among brain cell types and between those suffering from the disease and those who are healthy (HSCI 2016). It should be noted that, whether it be stem cells or other physical interventions, any such measures that fail to fully treat AD will add substantially to the overall cost of the disease.

Supplements and Homeopathic Medicines

A long-standing policy debate affecting AD treatment involves FDA regulation of the highly profitable enterprise of supplements and homeopathic drugs. All such products on the market fall within the definition of "drug" in the Food, Drug & Cosmetic Act of 1938 (FD&C Act). However, the FDA, without statutory authority, exempted homeopathic drugs from the regulatory scheme mandated by federal law. Likewise, supplements are regulated under the Dietary Supplement Health and Education Act of 1996 (DSHEA), which essentially removed them from FDA regulation as well. Although the Act was branded as being pro-consumer choice, it was blatantly pro-industry (Novella 2015). Without FDA control, the supplements industry can, in effect, make whatever claims it wants to without having to provide scientific evidence as long as they add a disclaimer noting the FDA has not reviewed the claims (see Box 3.3). These lax regulations essentially have created an opportunity to make fortunes off the placebo effect through aggressive marketing that supplements are "natural" and, thereby, safe and effective despite the fact they can have serious side effects, toxicity, and interactions (Bellamy 2015).

> **Box 3.3 Example of Disclaimer**
> *Health Disclaimer!* The information provided on this site should not be construed as personal medical advice or instruction. No action should be taken based solely on the contents of this site. Readers should consult appropriate health professionals on any matter relating to their health and well-being. The information and opinions provided here are believed to be accurate and sound, based on the best judgment available to the authors, but readers who fail to consult appropriate health authorities assume the risk of any injuries. The publisher is not responsible for errors or omissions (https:// www.amazon.com/Atlas-Natural-Cures-Glenn-Rothfeld/dp/ B01NCJ65HW).

According its proponents, homeopathy offers long-term therapies for people suffering from AD by removing blockages from blood vessels, improving blood circulation to the arteries and veins of the brain, and, thereby, slowing the degenerative process, reducing hormonal and neurotransmitter imbalances that lead to AD, and helping in repairing damaged brain cells. They contend that by acting on the sympathetic nervous system, homeopathic remedies also reduce anxiety associated with AD, help reduce mood fluctuations and depression, and restore cognitive functions. One site concludes that there are 49 medicines which give great relief in AD (http://homeopathictreatment4u.com/dementia.html).

The Society for Science-Based Medicine, however, contends that homeopathy is highly implausible, unsupported by scientific evidence, ineffective in treating illness, and, when relied upon instead of actual medicine, dangerous and even deadly (Bellamy 2015). They argue that, in accordance with its consumer protection mandate, the FDA should take immediate action to remedy this by requiring that all homeopathic products comply with the same statutes and regulations as other drugs, as is done in other countries. For example, assessments by the Australian National Health and Medical Research Council, the Swiss Federal Health Office, and the British House of Commons Science and Technology

Committee have all concluded that homeopathy is ineffective and have recommended against the practice receiving any further funding. The latter concluded: "In our view, the systematic reviews and meta-analyses conclusively demonstrate that homeopathic products perform no better than placebos. We could find no support from independent experts for the idea that there is good evidence for the efficacy of homeopathy." Furthermore, the British NHS recently announced a ban on the provision of homeopathic medicine because it is "a misuse of resources."

Traditional Chinese medicine (TCM) has been practiced in Chinese health care for more than 2000 years. Recently, researchers have isolated many unique compounds from herbs, some of which might improve AD with fewer side effects than conventional drugs. Wu et al. (2011) summarize research progress on six herbs for AD therapy and assess their possible pharmacological actions in alleviating dementia. They include: *Huperzia serrata*; plants belonging to the Amaryllidaceae family, which have been approved by the Chinese FDA and the US FDA for the treatment of mild to moderate AD; *Ginkgo biloba L*; *Uncaria rhynchophylla Havil*; *P tenuifolia Willdenow*, one of the most frequently used medicinal herbs for memory loss; and *Salvia officinalis L*, which has been found to reverse D-galactose-induced learning and memory impairment. Some active extracts or components from herbs are highly potent and multi-targeted with low toxicity for the treatment of AD. Although the underlying molecular mechanisms have not been fully elucidated, or their efficacy proven, proponents regard these herbs as promising sources of potential anti-AD drugs (Wu et al. 2011).

Regulating Natural Supplements

Although there is little to stop businesses from selling supposed remedies, no matter how dubious they are, recently, the United States appears to be moving toward closer regulation of the supplements industry. The FDA initiated a review of its regulation of homeopathy and has targeted regulation of the term "natural," while the Federal Trade Commission is reviewing the claims made by the homeopathy industry. Similarly, in 2015, the New York State Attorney General's office filed a cease-and-desist order against large pharmacy chains, to stop selling numerous herbal supplements that were found not to contain the ingredients on the label. Also, at the federal level, the Department of Justice has become involved in filing an indictment against OxyElite Pro Advanced Formula in late 2013, after it was associated with a rash of liver injuries with several users needing transplants (Novella 2015).

It is important to regulate health care products in the free market because it is not possible for consumers to evaluate long-term effects of products and services, especially where all product effects are obscured by placebo effects. Consumers cannot reasonably rely on the ads or on their own anecdotal experience. They need to be informed by scientific evidence that will not be generated and evaluated unless regulations compel it. These alternative drugs should be regulated as drugs, not food or vitamins. Moreover, the industry needs to be carefully monitored for quality control, transparency, and accuracy in labeling. Ironically, the public assumes this already exists and has no idea that they are at the mercy of the supplement industry's self-regulation.

SELECTED APPROACHES FOR TREATING ALZHEIMER'S

This section offers examples of recent studies using diverse approaches to AD treatment that are to some extent based on the use of nutrients. No attempt is made here to judge the veracity of the claims made by each, although in several cases, it should be obvious to the reader. Chapter 5 examines the evidence of potential preventive strategies in more detail.

Souvenaid

One study from Massachusetts Institute of Technology (MIT) announced that nutritional supplement sold over the counter in 15, mostly European, countries, although not the United States, can improve memory in patients with early AD (Trafton 2012). The supplement mixture Souvenaid contains three naturally occurring dietary compounds: choline, uridine, and the omega-3 fatty acid DHA, all of which are precursors to the lipid molecules that, along with specific proteins, make up brain-cell membranes that form synapses. Purportedly, Souvenaid can slow or reverse the loss of synapses leading to memory loss and other cognitive impairments of AD, but to be effective, all three compounds must be administered simultaneously. European clinical trials sponsored by Nutricia, which holds the exclusive license on the MIT patent, involved patients with mild AD.

The first trial found that 40 percent of patients who drank Souvenaid improved in a test of verbal memory, compared to 24 percent of those given the placebo. It also found that the supplement cocktail does not work in patients with more advanced AD, most likely because they have already lost too many neurons and are unable to form new synapses. A second six-month trial found that all subjects improved their verbal-memory performance for the first three months, but the placebo patients deteriorated during the following three months, while the Souvenaid patients continued to improve. At the 14th International Athens/Springfield Symposium on Advances in Alzheimer Therapy in 2016, researchers associated with the Souvenaid program presented their latest results (Zakaib 2016). They argued that, while a clinical trial funded by the European Union found no significant benefit on a composite measure of cognition, in a subset of trial participants at the earliest stages of pro-dromal AD, hippocampal volume increased and after two years, it had atrophied 39 percent more in the placebo than the treatment group. Co-author Pieter Jelle Visser suggests that Souvenaid could be of some benefit early in the disease when damage to the synapses is still limited, but that more data and replication are needed before routine treatment is recommended (quoted in Zakaib 2016).

Metabolic Enhancement for Neurodegeneration (MEND).

In 2014, a claim of the first reversal of cognitive decline in patients with early AD or its precursors was published (Bredesen 2014). The University of California-Los Angeles-based, personalized and inclusive program to reverse memory loss involved a small sample of patients who made dramatic lifestyle changes. The study was the first to suggest that memory loss in AD patients can be reversed, and improvement sustained. It entailed a complex, 36-point therapeutic program involving comprehensive diet changes, brain stimulation, exercise, sleep optimization, selected pharmaceuticals, and vitamins as well as multiple other steps that affect neural chemistry. Within six months, nine patients saw a noticeable restitution of memory, while one in the late stages of AD showed none. "Sustained and marked" improvements lasted up to two and one-half years from initial treatment, suggesting that, at least in the early stages, cognitive decline may be driven largely by metabolic processes.

According to Bredesen et al. (2016), it is possible that a multiple-component system approach, like that used for other chronic illnesses, which addresses numerous targets within the network underlying AD, works in an additive or synergistic way. His team found evidence that AD stems from an imbalance in nerve cell signaling. In the normal brain, specific signals foster nerve connections and memory making, while balancing signals support memory loss, allowing irrelevant information to be forgotten. But in people with AD, the balance of these opposing signals is disturbed, nerve connections are suppressed, and memories are lost. MEND is tailored to each patient, based on extensive testing to determine what is affecting the brain's plasticity signaling network. For example, components of the program for one early-stage AD patient included:

- eliminating all simple carbohydrates, gluten, and processed food from the diet, and eating more vegetables, fruits, and non-farmed fish
- meditating twice a day and practicing yoga to reduce stress
- sleeping seven to eight hours per night
- taking melatonin, methylcobalamin, vitamin D3, fish oil, and coenzyme Q10 each day
- optimizing oral hygiene using an electric flosser and toothbrush
- using hormone replacement therapy
- fasting a minimum of 12 hours between dinner and breakfast and a minimum of three hours between dinner and bedtime
- exercising for a minimum of 30 minutes, four to six days per week

Bredesen et al. (2016) contend that the program's only downside is its complexity and the responsibility it places on patients and carers to follow it. Despite this, the authors argue that memory loss might be reversed, and improvement sustained, with this program.

Ketones, Coconut Oil, and Ketone Ester

As noted in Chap. 1, one theory posits that a major feature of AD is progressive insulin deficiency and insulin resistance and that AD patients display a striking decrease in glucose use in certain brain areas that can originate up to 20 years before perceptible symptoms. Deprived of their main energy source, neurons can suffer irreparable damage. A compound called AC-1202 (medium chain triglyceride, or MCT, oil derived from coconut oil and sold in natural food stores since the 1960s) purportedly can provide glucose-deprived neurons with an alternative energy source known as ketone bodies, reverse problems of glucose transport common in AD, and mitigate memory problems and other functional losses (Newport 2011). The inventor of AC-1202 claims that mild ketosis produced by ingesting MCT improved the cognitive ability of a "significant number" of AD patients who exhibited little disease progression after six months (Newport 2011: 60).

Veech (2004), however, argues that MCT oil cannot work because the blood levels are only one-tenth those needed for transfer to the brain, and recommends using a ketone ester, which he synthesizes, instead as soon after a predisposition or genetic marker to AD is found. According to Veech, ketones share many of the same effects as insulin in the brain and can provide fuel to the mitochondria, which then increase the production of the metabolites needed to make ATP. In addition, ketone bodies can reduce damage to the mitochondria from free radicals. He suggests that with the introduction of ketones in the body some repair and reversal could occur in AD, since ketone bodies have been shown to increase the neurite outgrowths in hippocampal cells (Veech 2004). Allegedly, ketones also can stimulate the growth and survival of neurons as well as the axons and dendrites, thereby increasing the synapses among brain cells.

The ICT Protocol

The most ubiquitous entrepreneur of a cure to AD is a Dr. Glenn Rothfeld whose presence on the Internet is imposing and imaginative. According to his research assistant Christine O'Brien at the Institute of Natural Healing or the Rothfeld Center for Integrative Medicine, evidence has emerged that for over three years, researchers funded by the US government have been secretly reversing AD in their patients through "stunning transformations" that some doctors have called a cure. As "proof," they offer cases like Tom, a 69-year-old business owner who could not remember the names and faces of the people who worked for him. Brain scans showed clear evidence of AD and things were rapidly deteriorating. But just a few short months of this treatment *completely reversed his symptoms.* Medically speaking, his AD was cured. The "miracle" treatment is based on something called the ICT protocol. It is found in a book called *81 Natural Cures for Cancer, Diabetes, Alzheimer's and More,* that the doctor "generously" offers for free, although they have a *very* limited number of copies.

The ICT protocol is based on the presumption that the buildup of beta-amyloid plaques is essentially the final stage of the process, not the cause of AD. In other words, plaque is really a late-stage symptom of a deeper problem, which according to Rothfeld is starvation of brain cells. Our brain needs the right fuel to run properly, a fuel composed of highly specialized forms of nutrients like glucose, B-vitamins, choline, and phosphorous. When we are young, our digestion works well enough that we can get these critical nutrients from normal diets, but as we age it gets harder to absorb the nutrients. Since brain cells cannot work without them, they suffer the most, in effect starving to death. The ICT protocol triggers powerful transformations in AD patients because it is a super-nutrient cocktail designed to feed one's starving brain. The only revealed ingredient in the ad for the protocol is MCTs which were also a key part of the ketone treatment. With a regular dose of MCTs, brain cells have a new stream of energy at their disposal. Although MCTs alone may be powerful enough to reverse mild cases of mental decline, when combined with the other ingredients in the ICT protocol, the results are "downright incredible," according to the ad.

But, one might ask, if the ICT protocol works so well, why are not doctors everywhere recommending it to their patients. The answer for Dr. Rothfeld is a massive political conspiracy:

Well, I'm afraid the mainstream, liberal establishment can't let that happen. In June of 2010, President Obama publicly declared war on Alzheimer's disease. That's when he signed a bill called the National Alzheimer's Project Act (NAPA) into law. It involved millions in funding, and a green light for hundreds of new studies…It was great PR for Obama. Bumped up his approval ratings for a little while. But actually curing the disease? That was NEVER part of plan. See, NAPA—like all Big Government's "wars on disease"—was really just a handout to Big Pharma…You see, by creating programs like NAPA, the government gets to control the flow of money used for research. Then they funnel that money into research that they KNOW will never lead to a cure. For Alzheimer's disease, that means lots of studies on new prescription drugs, even though…Billions of dollars and decades of research into prescription Alzheimer's drugs have completely FAILED to slow the disease, let alone cure it! (The Vitamin Cocktail That Saves Your Mind and Wards off Dementia, https://www.institutefornaturalhealing.com/2013/05/the-vitamin-cocktail-that-saves-your-mind-and-wards-off-dementia/)

Antioxidants

Another pervasive presence on the Internet is Dr. Russell Blaylock, who purportedly spent his medical career as a celebrated neurosurgeon. But after seeing how often conventional medicine failed people, he spent decades studying the research on specific nutrients and other natural remedies and turned toward the use of nutrition in healing and wellness. Blaylock considers inflammation to be the "ground zero" of all health concerns including AD. To that end, he developed ADVANCIN™, an exclusive formula that contains a "proprietary blend of eight antioxidants and potent nutrients that work together to fight inflammation, provide antioxidant support, and promote the health of all organs." This "comprehensive and supercharged" ADVANCIN formula promotes proper inflammatory response throughout the body, fights free radical damage at the cellular level, may help support normal blood flow and fight premature aging related to oxidative stress, supports heart and brain health, and helps support healthy lipid levels. Unlike the secret ICT protocol, the eight ingredients ADVANCIN are listed: vitamin C; hesperidin; chamomile extract (apigenin); luteolin; bromelain; quercetin; resveratrol; and green tea.

> And here's the best news…Try ADVANCIN for 30 Days at No Charge with This Special Offer. Dr. Blaylock is confident in the benefits of ADVANCIN. So he was able to make special arrangements with the supplier, Medix Select, to reserve a bottle in your name. It's true…We've agreed to send you a 30-day trial supply at no charge. You cover only a $4.95 S&H fee. https://w3.medixselect.com/MedixTV/LP/Advancin-Urgent-Health-Alert?src=L3112&ns_mail_uid=96467334&ns_mail_job=1758878_10182017&s=al&dkt_nbr=010102oh89uj

Similarly, Blalock advertises a product called Cresceo that comprises five ingredients that "offer natural support for brain function, cognition, and memory" including: ginkgo biloba; bacopa monnieri (the Cresceo formula gives you 300 mg daily—the optimal dosage suggested by research); phosphatidylserine (Cresceo contains a proprietary form called SerinAid 50P to reduce age-related cognitive decline by supporting key brain functions); huperzine-A; and DMAE (dimethylaminoethanol) to speed up the brain's synthesis and turnover of the neurotransmitter acetylcholine and reduce cell membrane damage. The reader is invited to try Cresceo for 30 days as part of a risk-free trial offer.

SUMMARY

Commercialization and unregulated opportunities to profit from an illness are an issue with all diseases and conditions, but AD is even more problematic because the fear of dementia, exacerbated by the lack of proven treatment options, opens it up to less than scrupulous merchants of medicine. "Though dealing with AD can be frightening, one must be careful. Scared people are also vulnerable people. Though taking advantage of the vulnerable is as despicable as it sounds, one must play it safe. Where there is a dollar to be earned … you can bet that someone will swoop in for that money" (The Thought Zone 2017). As illustrated by the examples here, there are degrees of misrepresentation, deception, and duplicity involved. Marketing strategies range from a subtle stretching of the scientific evidence to fit one's purpose or downright fraud and the lines between are often hazy.

References

Bellamy, J. (2015) "Society for Science-Based Medicine: Comment to FDA on homeopathic drug regulation." https://sciencebasedmedicine.org/society-for-science-based-medicine-comment-to-fda-on-homeopathic-drug-regulation/.

Blank, R.H. (2015) *Cognitive Enhancement: Social and Public Policy Issues.* London: Palgrave Press.

Boggio, P.S., L.P. Khoury, D.C. Martins, O.E. Martins et al. (2009) "Temporal cortex direct current stimulation enhances performance on a visual recognition memory task in Alzheimer disease." *Journal of Neurology and Neurosurgery Psychiatry* 80 (4): 444–47.

Boot, W.R. and A.F. Kramer (2014) "The brain-games conundrum: Does cognitive training really sharpen the mind?" Cerebrum. http://dana.org/Cerebrum/2014/The_Brain-ames_Conundrum_Does_Cognitive_Training_Really_Sharpen_the_Mind_/.

Bredesen, D.E. (2014) "Reversal of cognitive decline: A novel therapeutic program." *Aging* 6 (9): 707–17.

Bredesen, D.E., E.C. Amos, J. Canick, M. Ackerley et al. (2016) "Reversal of cognitive decline in Alzheimer's disease." *Aging* 8 (6): 1250–58.

Conrad, P. and A. Horwitz (2013) "Marketing of neuropsychiatric illness and enhancement." In A. Chatterjee and M.J. Farah, eds., *Neuroethics in Practice: Medicine, Mind, and Society.* New York: Oxford University Press, pp. 46–56.

Corbett, A., A.M. Owen, A. Hampshire, J. Grahn et al. (2015) "The effect of an online cognitive training package in healthy older adults: An online randomized controlled trial." *Journal of the American Medical Directors Association* 16: 990–97.

Cote, D.J., A.L. Bredenoord, T.R. Smith, M. Ammirati et al. (2017) "Ethical clinical translation of stem cell interventions for neurologic disease." *Neurology* 88 (3): 322–28.

Cotelli, M., R. Manenti, M. Brambilla, M. Petesi et al. (2014) "Anodal tDCS during face-name associations memory training in Alzheimer's patients." *Frontiers in Aging Neuroscience.* https://doi.org/10.3389/fnagi.2014.00038

Coveney, C., J. Gabe and S. Williams (2011) "The sociology of cognitive enhancement: Medicalisation and beyond." *Health Sociology Review* 20 (4): 381–93.

Cummings, J., G. Lee, T. Mortsdorf, A. Ritter and K. Zhong (2017) "Alzheimer's disease drug development pipeline: 2017." *Alzheimer's & Dementia: Translational Research & Clinical Interventions* 3 (3): 367–84.

de Boer, M.E., C.M.P.M. Hertogh, R. Droes et al. (2007) "Suffering from dementia: The patient's perspective." *International Psychogeriatrics* 19 (6): 1021–39.

Drakos, A. (2015) "tDCS and Alzheimer's Disease." *Brainstorm Blog.* http://www.tdcsbrainstorm.com/brainstormblog/tdcs-and-alzheimers-disease.

Draper, B., C. Peisaha, J. Snowdon and H. Brodaty (2010) "Early dementia diagnosis and the risk of suicide and euthanasia." *Alzheimer's and Dementia* 6: 75–82.

Elder, G.J. and J-P. Taylor (2014) "Transcranial magnetic stimulation and transcranial direct current stimulation: Treatments for cognitive and neuropsychiatric symptoms in the neurodegenerative dementias?" *Alzheimer's Research and Therapy* 6: 74–85.

Ferrucci, R., F. Mameli, I. Guidi, S. Mrakic-Sposta et al. (2008) "Transcranial direct current stimulation improves recognition memory in Alzheimer disease." *Neurology* 71 (7): 493–98.

Garrett, M.D. (2013) "Fear of dementia: The emerging fear in America." *Psychology Today.* https://www.psychologytoday.com/blog/iage/201305/fear-dementia.

Ghoravshi, A. (2014) "Brain games exploit anxieties about memory loss for profit." *The Guardian.* http://www.theguardian.com/science/2014/oct/23/brain-games-memory-loss-open-letter#sthash.CSyjdlU2.dpuf.

Gilbert, F. and D. Ovadia (2011) "Deep brain stimulation in the media: Over-optimistic portrayals call for a new strategy involving journalists and scientists in ethical debates." *Frontiers in Integrative Neuroscience* 5: 16. https://doi.org/10.3389/fnint.2011.00016.

Gordon, M. (2015) "Alzheimer's disease, media representations and the politics of euthanasia: Constructing risk and selling death in an ageing society by Megan-Jane Johnstone (review)." *Canadian Journal on Aging/La Revue canadienne du vieillissement* 34 (2): 258–60.

Gullettemay, M.M. (2011) "Our irrational fear of forgetting." *New York Times.* http://www.nytimes.com/2011/05/22/opinion/22gullette.html.

Hanrahan, D. (2013) "Ethical issues surrounding direct-to-consumer advertising of neurotechnology." *Ethics in Biology, Engineering and Medicine: An International Journal:* 173–84. https://doi.org/10.1615/EthicsBiologyEngMed.2013007012.

Harvard Stem Cell Institute (2016) http://hsci.harvard.edu/alzheimers-disease-0.

Hertogh, C.M.P.M. (2005) "End-of-life care and medical decision making in patients with dementia." In A. Burns, ed., *Standards in Dementia Care: European Dementia Consensus Network (EDCON)*. New York: Taylor & Francis, pp. 339–54.

Hohenfeld, C., N. Nellessen, I. Dogan, H. Kuhn et al. (2017) "Cognitive improvement and brain changes after real-time functional MRI: Neurofeedback training in healthy elderly and prodromal Alzheimer's disease." *Frontiers in Neurology* 8: 384. https://doi.org/10.3389/fneur.2017.00384.

Honig, L.S., B. Vellas, M. Woodward, M. Boada et al. (2018) "Trial of solanezumab for mild dementia due to Alzheimer's disease." *New England Journal of Medicine* 378 (4): 321–30.

Hsieh, E. (2015) "On the horizon: A magnetic zap that strengthens memory." *Scientific American Mind* 26 (3): 15. https://doi.org/10.1038/scientificamericanmind0515-15a.

Humphreys, G. (2009) "Direct-to-consumer advertising under fire." *Bulletin of the World Health Organization* 87: 576–77.

Kang, J.M., B.K. Yeon, S.J. Cho and Y.H. Suh (2016) "Stem cell therapy for Alzheimer's disease: A review of recent clinical trials." *Journal of Alzheimer's Disease* 54 (3): 879–89.

Kunkle, F. (2015) "Alzheimer's spurs the fearful to change their lives to delay it." *Washington Post*. https://www.washingtonpost.com/local/social-issues/fear-of-alzheimers-is-everywhere-but-its-spurring-some-people-to-change-their-lives-for-the-better/2015/07/04/c0600046-192a-11e5-93b7-5ed-dc056ad8a_story.html.

Laxton, A.W. and A.M. Lozano (2013) "Deep brain stimulation for the treatment of Alzheimer's disease and dementias." *World Neurosurgery* 80 (3–4): S28.e1–S28.e8.

Laxton, A.W., D.F. Tang-Wai, M.P. McAndrews et al. (2010) "A phase 1 trial of deep brain stimulation of memory circuits in Alzheimer's disease." *Annals of Neurology* 68 (4): 521–34.

Le Couteur, D.G., B. Bateman and C. Brayne (2018) "Dalopirdine: Another disappointment for people with dementia." *British Medical Journal* 360: k753.

Lozano, A.M., L. Fosdick, M.M. Chakravarty, J-M. Leoutsakos et al. (2016) "A phase II study of fornix deep brain stimulation in mild Alzheimer's disease." *Journal of Alzheimer's Disease* 54 (2): 777–87.

Marceglia, S., S. Mrakic-Sposta, M. Rosa, R. Ferrucci, F. Mameli et al. (2016) "Transcranial direct current stimulation modulates cortical neuronal activity in Alzheimer's disease." *Frontiers in Neuroscience* 10: 134. https://doi.org/10.3389/fnins.2016.00134.

Maslen, H., T. Douglas, R. Cohen Kadosh, N. Levy and J. Savulescu (2014) "The regulation of cognitive enhancement devices: Extending the medical model." *Journal of Law and the Biosciences* 1: 68–93.

Max Planck Institute for Human Development and Stanford Center on Longevity (2014) "A consensus on the brain training industry from the scientific community." http://longevity.stanford.edu/a-consensus-on-the-brain-training-industry-from-the-scientific-community-2/.

Meinzer, M., R. Lindenberg, M.T. Phan, L. Ulm et al. (2015) "Transcranial direct current stimulation in mild cognitive impairment: Behavioral effects and neural mechanisms." *Alzheimer's and Dementia* 11 (9): 1032–40.

Mrakic-Sposta, S., M. Rosa, R. Ferrucci, F. Mameli et al. (2016) "Transcranial direct current stimulation modulates cortical neuronal activity in Alzheimer's disease." *Frontiers in Neuroscience* 10: 134. https://doi.org/10.3389/fnins.2016.00134.

Newport, M.T. (2011) *Alzheimer's Disease: What if There Was a Cure? The story of Ketones*. Laguna Beach, CA: Basic Health Publications.

Novacic, I. (2016) "Alzheimer's patients test deep brain stimulation to help boost memory." http://www.cbsnews.com/news/for-alzheimers-patients-new-clinical-trial-could-help-stimulate-memory/.

Novella, S. (2015) "US Department of Justice goes after supplements." https://sciencebasedmedicine.org/us-department-of-justice-goes-after-supplements/.

Owen, A.M., A. Hampshire, J.A. Grahn, R. Stenton, S. Dajani, A.S. Burns et al. (2010) "Putting brain training to the test." *Nature* 465 (7299): 775–78.

Palmour, N. and E. Racine (2011) "Direct-to-consumer marketing of dietary supplements for dementia: An example of unhealthy commerce of neuroscience." *AJOB Neuroscience* 2 (4): 30–33.

Racine, E., H.A. van der Loos and J. Illes (2007) "Internet marketing of neuroproducts: New practices and healthcare policy challenges." *Cambridge Quarterly of Healthcare Ethics* 16 (2): 181–94.

Redick, T.S., Z. Shipstead, T.L. Harrison, K.L. Hicks et al. (2013) "No evidence of intelligence improvement after working memory training: A randomized, placebo-controlled study." *Journal of Experimental Psychology: General* 142 (2): 359–79.

Research!America Health Poll (2006) "Top concerns about aging: Failing health, mental ability." http://www.researchamerica.org/sites/default/files/uploads/poll2006mentalhealth.pdf.

Sabat, S.R. (2018) *Alzheimer's Disease and Dementia: What Everyone Needs to Know*. Oxford: Oxford University Press.

Stem Cell Therapy Plus (2016) http://www.stemcelltherapyplus.com/.

StemGenex (2016) "Can stem cell therapy help patients with Alzheimer's disease?" https://stemgenex.com/studies/alzheimers-stem-cell-studies/?utm_source=bing&utm_medium=cpc&utm_campaign=Alzheimer%27s&utm_content=Stem%20Cell&utm_term=%2Balzheimers%20%2BStem%20%2BCell.

Sulzer, J., S. Haller, F. Scharnowski, N. Weiskopf et al. (2013) "Real-time fMRI neurofeedback: Progress and challenges." *Neuroimage* 76: 386–99.

Telegraph (2014) "Older people are more scared of dementia than cancer, poll finds." http://www.telegraph.co.uk/news/health/elder/11008905/Older-people-are-more-scared-of-dementia-than-cancer-poll-finds.html.

The Thought Zone (2017) "The cure to dementia: A beverage?" https://mbman.wordpress.com/2017/06/01/the-cure-to-dementia-a-beverage/.

Thraves, L. (2015) "Stem cell research." https://www.alzheimers.org.uk/site/scripts/documents_info.php?documentID=430.

Trafton, A. (2012) "In clinical trial, mixture developed at MIT appears to help overcome loss of connections between brain cells. Nutrient mixture improves memory in patients with early Alzheimer's." *MIT News.* http://news.mit.edu/2012/alzheimers-nutrient-mixture-0709.

Veech, R.L. (2004) "The therapeutic implications of ketone bodies: The effects of ketone bodies in pathological conditions: Ketosis, ketogenic diet, redox states, insulin resistance, and mitochondrial metabolism." *Prostaglandins, Leukotrienes and Essential Fatty Acids* 70 (3): 309–19.

Whitehouse, P.J. and D. George (2008) *The Myth of Alzheimer's.* New York: St. Martin's Press.

Wu, T-Y., C-P. Chen and T-R. Jinn (2011) "Traditional Chinese medicines and Alzheimer's disease." *Taiwanese Journal of Obstetrics & Gynecology* 50: e131–e135.

Yuan, H., S. Tabarak, Jing Yu and Xu Lei (2015) "Transcranial direct current stimulation in patients with Alzheimer's disease: Challenges and responses." *ADMET & DMPK* 3 (3): 235–41.

Zakaib, G.D. (2016) "Souvenaid trial missed primary, partially met secondary endpoints." http://www.alzforum.org/news/conference-coverage/souvenaid-trial-missed-primary-partially-met-secondary-endpoints.

CHAPTER 4

Caregivers, Long-Term Care, and Social Health

Abstract Alzheimer's disease is the costliest disease in large part because of its long duration of disability and resulting need for labor-intensive long-term care (LTC). This chapter examines both informal and formal caregivers and the heavy burden placed on families, primarily women. It analyzes the tension between home versus institutional care and recent policy attempts to strengthen LTC services. The chapter then analyzes the emerging emphasis on the social health of AD patients and summarizes research across many disciplines in developing new care approaches.

Keywords Long-term care for AD patients • Caretakers • Burden of Alzheimer's on families • Social health of AD patients

AD is the costliest disease in large part because of its long duration of disability and resulting need for labor-intensive LTC. This chapter examines both informal and formal caregivers and the heavy burden placed on families, primarily women. It analyzes the tension between home versus institutional care and recent policy attempts to strengthen LTC services. Finally, it analyzes the emerging emphasis on the social health of AD patients and summarizes research across many disciplines for developing new care approaches.

© The Author(s) 2019
R. H. Blank, *Social & Public Policy of Alzheimer's Disease in the United States*, https://doi.org/10.1007/978-981-13-0656-3_4

LTC comprises a broad range of day-to-day help needed by people with chronic conditions, disabilities, or frailty. This can include personal care (bathing, dressing, toileting); complex care (wound care); help with housekeeping, transportation, paying bills, and meals; and other ongoing social services. The former tasks are often designated as activities of daily living (ADLs) while those such as managing medications or finances are termed instrumental activities of daily living (IADLs). LTC may be provided in one's home, an assisted living or other supportive housing setting, nursing facilities, or in integrated settings that provide both health care and supportive services.

AD presents distinctive issues within LTC because of its high prevalence, progressive nature, and long duration. Moreover, demographic trends suggest that the current heavy reliance on family caregiving is unsustainable. As the median age of the population trends upward, the imbalance between the number of people needing care and those available to deliver it will widen. Greater rates of childlessness, smaller and more geographically dispersed families, and increasing participation of women in the labor force pose threats to the availability of family caregivers to meet the needs of the growing number of older Americans. Moreover, advances in medicine that have extended life expectancy have increased the duration, complexity, and technical difficulty of care. The AARP Public Policy Institute estimates that the ratio of caregivers aged 45–64 to each person aged 80 and older who needs LTC will decline from 7:1 in 2010 to less than 3:1 in 2050 (Redfoot et al. 2013).

AD LTC is also problematic because of its effects on behavior and ability to self-manage care due to impaired cognitive and decision-making capabilities, risk of abuse, high rate of comorbid health conditions, heavy reliance on and resulting health impacts on caregivers, and higher costs associated with LTC compared to other chronic conditions. Furthermore, AD patients experience transitions across the progressive stages, but the settings and facilities that provide LTC during these transitions frequently operate in isolation with little coordination across data systems (Shih et al. 2014).

An important trend in the delivery of LTC services over the past decades has been a deliberate "rebalancing" of care away from institutional settings such as nursing homes and toward home- and community-based settings. This shift is reflected in the share of Medicaid spending for these services, which doubled between 1995 and 2011 and is growing at a much faster rate than spending on institutional services (Ng et al. 2014).

In 2013, home- and community-based services represented 51 percent of Medicaid spending on long-term services and supports, with the remaining 49 percent for institutional care. Home care traverses the lines between health and social care and between formal and informal care. Although a critical area of health policy, it often is not fully integrated in the institutional fabric of health systems. Home care funding is typically highly mixed because funding from public sources is often insufficient and a large amount of services is funded by out-of-pocket payments (Pavolini and Theobald 2015; Campbell et al. 2016).

THE INFORMAL LTC WORKFORCE

Historically, caring for ill family members was rarely viewed as a public issue because it was assumed to be a role of women within the extended family (Alzheimer's Association 2016). Until the mid-1990s, family care was often supplemented by paid help, but today shortages of formal care workers and/or inability to pay for adequate services leave many family caregivers with no alternative but to provide care themselves (Houser et al. 2010). Two-thirds of older people with disabilities who receive LTC at home get all their care from their family caregivers, mostly spouses and adult daughters. Another quarter (26 percent) receives some combination of family care and paid help while only 9 percent relies solely on paid help (Doty 2010). Another change is that in the past care was typically short term, because most people died from acute, rather than chronic, conditions such as AD. Moreover, the trend toward shorter hospital stays and increased demands and budget cuts for home- and community-based services place even more responsibilities and economic burdens on families.

Over 80 percent of the help provided to older adults in the United States comes from family members, friends, or other unpaid caregivers. In 2017, more than 16 million Americans provided about 18.4 billion hours of unpaid care to AD patients, worth $232 billion (Alzheimer's Association 2018). One AARP report estimated the economic value of family caregiving considerably higher at $450 billion based on 42.1 million caregivers aged 18 or older providing an average of 18.4 hours of care per week at an average value of $11.16 per hour (Feinberg et al. 2011). A longitudinal study of the monetary value of family caregiving for individuals with AD found that the overall value of daily family care increased 18 percent with each additional year of providing care, and that the value of daily care increased as the care recipient's cognitive abilities declined (Wolff et al. 2016). Without families' unpaid contributions, the health and LTC systems would be overwhelmed by the need for supportive services.

Caring for a spouse with AD is particularly stressful and is associated with depression, sleep problems, social isolation, mortality, and a greater risk of the caregiver developing dementia (Reinhard et al. 2014). It is estimated that at least 40 percent of family caregivers have clinically significant depression or anxiety while others exhibit less severe, but debilitating, psychological symptoms (Livingston et al. 2017). They also have poorer physical health, more work absences, and lower life quality than noncaregivers (Goren et al. 2016). They are more likely to have emergency department visits or hospitalization in the previous six months if taking care of individuals with heavy care needs (Schubert et al. 2008). Because caregivers often do not have free time for themselves, they frequently experience social isolation from a loss of social contacts. In turn, caregivers' health problems can affect their ward and wider society, if they lead to care breakdown and possible abuse (Gallagher et al. 2013).

Caring for an AD patient can also affect the caregiver's own work situation and retirement security. Almost 70 percent of report making work accommodations when work requirements come into conflict with caregiving tasks. One analysis estimates that the lifetime income-related losses sustained by family caregivers over age 50 who leave the workforce to care for a parent are $115,900 in wages, $137,980 in Social Security benefits, and at least $50,000 in pension benefits. These estimates range from a total of $283,716 for men to $324,044 for women, or $303,880 on average, in lost income and benefits over a lifetime (MetLife Mature Market Institute 2011). Assuming the role of caregiver for aging parents in midlife not only has a large economic impact on retirement, but also may substantially increase the risks of living in poverty and receiving public assistance in old age (Wakabayashi and Donato 2006).

Moreover, the economic impact extends beyond the caregivers. It is estimated that US businesses lose up to $33.6 billion per year in lost productivity from caregiving employees (MetLife 2010). These costs include those associated with replacing employees, absenteeism, workday distractions, supervisory time, and reductions in hours from full-time to part-time. Moreover, US employers were found to be paying about 8 percent more for the health care of employees with caregiving responsibilities compared to other employees, potentially costing them an additional $13.4 billion per year.

Based on nationwide poll of 3118 adults, including over 500 caregivers, the Shriver Report (2010) reveals the effect on women as caregivers, advocates, and people living with AD. According to the Report, women represent nearly two-thirds of all Americans with AD and comprise 60 percent of the unpaid caregivers. This means there are ten million women who either have AD or are caring for someone with it. Moreover, one-third have served in that role for over five years. Furthermore, one-third of the 6.7 million female caregivers are a part of the "sandwich generation" simultaneously caring for children and an adult with AD. The poll found that 64 percent reported that they had to arrive late, leave early, or ask for time off and most found it more difficult to get employer support for elder care than child care. It also found that 56 percent said that AD had strained their family's finances with an average cost of care of $56,800 annually with 60 percent, or $34,500, borne by the family themselves. Although the bulk of this ($27,200) is in the form of uncompensated care, out-of-pocket costs to families averaged $7259 per year for adult day care, assisted living, and paid companions or home health aides.

According to an AARP study (Keenan 2010), most caregivers are unprepared for the financial realities of LTC. Over half of have not planned for their own LTC needs, and 40 percent do not understand what it entails. Although over 80 percent know that one year in a nursing home is more expensive than four years of college, when asked about specific examples of care their estimates of costs vary widely. Moreover, only one-quarter is aware that Medicare does not cover these services because as AD progresses most care is not health care, but rather care dealing with ADLs. One has only two options to nursing homes: either continue with informal care, or use private funds to hire formal help. With home health aides costing an average of $21 an hour and assisted living facilities $38,000 a year, the latter is not a viable option for many families.

Effective interventions to reduce stress must be individually tailored, be multi-component, and focus on the capacity to make active, informed choices (Livingston et al. 2017). Education to increase knowledge about AD plays a necessary but not sufficient role in improving mental health (Corbett et al. 2012). Similarly, group behavioral therapy, support from trained family caregivers, group reminiscence therapy, counseling, and social support have not proven effective (Koivisto et al. 2016), although many novel interventions have been introduced. One of these, the STrAtegies for RelaTives (START) intervention, implemented in some centers in Britain, is a manual-based, eight-session therapy that includes planning for the future and allows the caregiver to work with a plan to select strategies they find most effective. START was found useful in preventing and treating depression and is cost-effective because it is delivered by supervised psychology graduates instead of clinical psychologists (Livingston et al. 2014).

In summary, informal caregiving is now recognized as a critical part of LTC care and services due to many converging factors including the aging population, the increasing prevalence of AD and other chronic conditions, critical shortages and costs in the formal care workforce, and the shift away from institutional care to more home care services, which, in any case, is what most older persons prefer. If informal caregivers were no longer available, the economic cost to the US health care and LTC systems would increase astronomically (Feinberg et al. 2011). Family caregiving also has been shown to help delay or prevent the use of nursing home care (Spillman and Long 2009). High levels of caregiver stress are a strong predictor of nursing home entry, thus reducing stress can reduce the rate of nursing home admission. Involving caregivers in discharge planning during transitions between hospital and home may not only improve quality of care, but also help to prevent hospital readmissions among Medicare beneficiaries (Naylor et al. 2011).

THE FORMAL LTC WORKFORCE

With respect to formal care, most who provide LTC services are direct care workers, including nursing aides, home health aides, and personal- or home-care aides (Shih et al. 2014). One significant gap in the LTC service workforce stems from the growing disparity between the demand for, and supply of, qualified, paid workers. This is exacerbated by high turnover and difficulty attracting qualified workers for low-paid caregiver jobs. Shortfalls in this workforce are often filled via the gray market of untrained helpers, leaving older adults vulnerable to poor or unregulated care. Furthermore, certification requirements for paraprofessional caregivers are nominal to non-existent in most states, and federal requirements are negligible, often less than two weeks of training (Shih et al. 2014). Not surprisingly, inadequate training for AD in the direct care workforce has been identified as a main contributor to poor quality of care, neglect, and abuse in some nursing homes (National Association of State Units on Aging 2005). This workforce would benefit substantially from in-depth training in how to manage behavioral symptoms related to AD but that requires time and money.

Despite the low pay of both institutional and home care formal caregivers, the costs of such care for persons with AD are high, and they increase sharply as cognitive impairment worsens. In 2012, the average annual cost of a private room in a nursing home in the United States was $81,030, a semi-private room $73,000, a licensed home health aide $43,472, homemaker services $41,184, a one-bedroom assisted living facility $39,600, and an adult day health center $15,860 (SCAN 2013). Special memory care locked-in facilities can exceed $100,000 per year. With respect to paid LTC services, Medicaid is the largest payer, funding about 62 percent, with the remainder funded out of pocket (22 percent), other private including insurance (12 percent) and other public (4 percent) (SCAN 2013). Medicaid can cover nursing home care and paid care provided in the home or community, as well as assistance with personal care, while Medicare finances only hospice costs and a portion of short-stay, post-acute care for beneficiaries (SCAN Foundation 2013). However, Medicaid eligibility rules in many states require that individuals have assets no greater than $2000, resulting in significant gaps in risk protection from high LTC costs.

People with substantial resources can plan early enough to buy private LTC insurance or pay out-of-pocket resources for financing, while lower-income individuals are covered through Medicaid, therefore leaving the middle-income population at greatest risk for significant and possibly catastrophic cost. Attempts to address this gap, such as the LTC State Partnership Program, available in 31 states to promote the purchase of private LTC coverage, never increased LTC coverage to the extent anticipated (Alper 2006). At the same time, the costs of LTC policies continue to rise. The average annual premium for an LTC insurance policy purchased in 2010 was $2255 for individuals aged 55–64, $2759 for those aged 65–69, and $3294 for those aged 70–74 (SCAN 2013).

CARE HOMES AND ASSISTED LIVING FACILITIES

Not all care homes offer specialist dementia services, despite about 80 percent of residents being affected (Lai et al. 2009), although recently dedicated memory care units have proliferated. Care homes vary widely in terms of organizational characteristics, processes such as access to specialized dementia care, case management, and palliative care, and structures of care such as hours of care provided per resident, level of expertise, and diversity of workforce (Zimmerman et al. 2013). They also differ in terms of practices such as anti-psychotic prescribing. Although those living in care homes usually have a lower quality of life than those at home (Beerens et al. 2013), because some experience more social support, reduced isolation, and improved care in the care home, their quality of life improves (Moyle and O'Dwyer 2012).

Assisted living, including extra-care sheltered housing, intermediate care housing, housing with care, or assisted living residences, is a progressively common option for those unable to live in their own home. Estimates indicate that 45–67 percent of residents of such facilities have AD, of whom more than half are moderate to severe with at least one neuropsychiatric symptom (Smith et al. 2008). Integration of AD services that incorporate person-centered care, activity, sensory stimulation, and monitoring of psychotropic medication can decrease agitation (Zimmerman et al. 2013). Interest in home-like residential care models and development of fit for the future residential settings is increasing. Examples include the Eden Alternative and other small-scale facilities that are specifically designed for people with AD (Verbeek et al. 2009). Some studies indicate that AD patients might benefit from these models as to their physical functioning; however, comparative-effectiveness and cost-effectiveness research is incomplete (Ausserhofer et al. 2016).

Many AD patients could benefit from the assisted living model, where they live independently in an apartment-like community and get assistance with meals, housekeeping, and some personal care, but, as with nursing homes, a large portion of the population that needs that level of care cannot afford it. Medicaid will cover assisted living in exceptional cases, but again only after the patient's assets are depleted. As a result, most nursing home residents who qualify for Medicaid must spend their Social Security and any other monthly income, except for a small personal needs allowance. Medicaid only makes up the difference if the nursing home resident cannot pay the full cost of care or has a financially dependent spouse.

ABUSE AND NEGLECT OF AD PATIENTS

One sensitive policy issue, often hidden, involves abuse or neglect of AD patients in either their homes or institutional care. Those with advanced stages of AD, especially, are vulnerable to abuse because of their isolation, reduced autonomy, complete dependence on caregivers, and problems communicating. Alleged abuses of patients in nursing homes are commonplace news stories, but similar abuse by families often goes undetected. Thus, while it is estimated that one-quarter of AD patients experience abuse, only a small proportion is ever reported (Livingston et al. 2017). One study found that between 27.9 and 62.3 percent of dementia patients face verbal abuse and 3.5–23.1 percent physical abuse (Dong et al. 2014).

Abuse can be verbal or psychological such as name calling, threatening, or humiliating, or physical that includes hitting or slapping as well as overzealous medication, restraint, or confinement arising from institutional policies or routines. Financial and sexual abuse involves inducing someone to enter into a financial or sexual transaction to which they unable to consent, while neglect involves failing to provide appropriate care or denying the necessities of life, such as adequate nutrition, sanitation, or heating. More than a third of family caregivers report behaving abusively toward their ward, although some of this can be reciprocal since those who are abusive themselves are most likely to be abused (Cooper et al. 2010). There is a fine line between proportionate self-defense and abuse, but laws should be in place that protect AD patients where possible.

Heightened concern about overuse of anti-psychotic drugs for AD patients in care facilities has led to decreased use and increased education and support of care home staff, although evidence of permanent effectiveness and sustainability is lacking. For instance, a study of care homes that already had a low frequency of anti-psychotic use found that reducing anti-psychotics, without adding other interventions for neuropsychiatric symptoms, is not helpful because these symptoms generally increase (Ballard et al. 2016). Successful implementation of any intervention requires substantial training and long-term supervision of care home staff, but this too can be costly (Rapaport et al. 2017).

Policy Developments in Long-Term Care

"Long-term care is arguably the largest unfunded health-related need we have in this country," according to aging expert R. Tamara Konetzka (quoted in Ramnarace 2010). Although a few countries have instituted universal LTC insurance, the United States displays a patchwork that varies widely from state to state. A recent attempt to initiate a public LTC program, the Community Living Assistance Services and Supports Act (CLASS Act) was enacted as Title VIII of the Patient Protection and

Affordable Care Act of 2010. It was meant to create a voluntary and public LTC insurance option administered by DHHS and funded by premiums voluntarily deducted from workers' pay checks. However, in 2011 the Obama Administration announced it was unworkable and would be not be implemented, and it was repealed in 2013.

One policy option that has been used in some countries is to compensate informal caregivers, although, in most cases, the payments are token amounts (Burau et al. 2007). For instance, the Netherlands adopted a systematic approach with financial support for informal caregivers as part of the introduction of a "personal budget" (a cash benefit) in 1995. Similarly, in Germany the introduction of LTC insurance extended the commitment to unpaid informal care (Theobald and Hampel 2013). Australia, too, has a long tradition of public support for family caregivers and the Department of Families, Community Services and Indigenous Affairs administers two allowances for them. These payments, theoretically, can help ease the burden on those who must take a leave of absence from their jobs, lose job benefits, or choose early retirement because of their responsibilities. Other ideas include giving caregivers more support services, such as easier access to adult day care, so they can remain in the workforce longer.

For the last decade, the AARP has published the Long-Term Services and Supports (LTSS) State Scorecard, a compilation of state data and analysis (Reinhard et al. 2014). The scorecard ranks the states on their performance for creating high-quality systems of care for older adults and people with physical disabilities and their family caregivers. It provides comparable state data to benchmark performance, measure progress, identify areas for improvement, and improve the lives of LTC users. In 2017, the AARP updated the LTSS Scorecard, concluding that overall the states have made incremental improvements since 2014, but that the pace of change is "slow and uneven" even though many state budgets are now healthier (Eisenberg 2017). The scorecard analyzes data in five categories of LTSS: affordability and access; choice of setting and provider; quality of life and care; support for family caregivers; and effective transitions. In 2017, no state was in the top quartile in every category. The top-ranking states were Washington, Minnesota, Vermont, Oregon, and Alaska while the lowest were Indiana, Kentucky, Alabama, Mississippi, and Tennessee.

Although most states showed no change in the affordability and access category, with nursing homes often costing more than $90,000 a year and a home health aide running $30,000 annually, not all of AARP's LTC news in 2017 was bad. For instance, 48 states reduced the use of anti-psychotic medications for nursing home residents. This was the result of action by the federal government to begin regulating their use and grading nursing homes on the percent of dementia patients receiving anti-psychotic medications in Medicare's Nursing Home Compare online tool. In addition, 39 states passed the CARE Act (Caregiver Advise, Record, Enable), a law that requires hospitals to record the name of any family caregiver on the AD patient's medical record, inform them when the patient is to be discharged, and provide education and instruction of medical tasks they will need to perform for the patient at home. AARP did again find major disparities among the states in certain categories of LTSS, for instance, the portion of Medicaid and state funding for home- and community-based services, which has been growing overall, but at a rate that will take 51 years for the average of the bottom five states to reach the level of the top five states.

Long-Term Care Policy Initiatives

As noted earlier, a few countries have established LTC insurance plans including Germany (Theobald and Ozanne 2016) and Japan (Campbell et al. 2016). Moreover, in 2008, Taiwan initiated a ten-year LTC plan to create a more integrated service delivery system and lay a foundation for the establishment of an LTC insurance program (Nadash and Shih 2012). As might be expected, in the United States public sources of funding for LTC remain marginal, commonly means-tested, and highly disjointed across states. According to a comprehensive study of LTC for the RAND Corporation (Shih et al. 2014), there remain severe challenges in LTC service delivery in the United States. While LTC for AD varies from state to state, overall publicly financed formal home- or community-based services remain unaffordable for middle-income families who must pay for these services out of pocket due to Medicaid eligibility requirements.

Building on the US DHHS's National Plan to Address Alzheimer's Disease (2014) and the Commission on Long-Term Care's Report to Congress (2013) that outlined national plans for strengthening LTC services and AD care, RAND provided a blueprint that address challenges with: stigma and early detection of signs and symptoms of AD that affect downstream access to quality care; inadequate access to, and measurement of, quality LTC services; fragmented delivery systems that especially affect persons with AD because of the reliance on services both outside and inside the traditional health care system; insufficient resource-finding infrastructure, employer programs, and financial resources to support family carers; and inadequate public and private options to help individuals and their families deal with the potentially devastating costs associated with LTC services. Instead of relying on a top-down approach in which federal agencies set priorities and implement the strategies, RAND identified options through engagement with a range of stakeholders from federal, state, and local levels, including patients, the public, purchasers, formal and informal providers, public and private payers, policy makers, and researchers (Shih et al. 2014).

From 38 policy options identified by various stakeholders, RAND researchers evaluated these options against pre-specified criteria and produced a list of 25 high-impact policy options and research directions to help policy makers improve the AD LTC delivery system, workforce, and financing. These policy options were summarized into five objectives to: (1) increase public awareness of AD to reduce stigma and promote earlier detection; (2) improve access to and use of LTC; (3) promote high-quality, person- and caregiver-centered care; (4) provide better support for families of people with AD; and (5) reduce the burden of LTC costs on individuals and families. Although they recommended that these policy options be considered for implementation immediately, they admitted that many options cannot be pursued in isolation and must be bundled to optimize successful implementation and maximum impact on access, quality, and utilization of LTC (Shih et al. 2014). Moreover, some recommendations are likely to face significant legal, political, and operational obstacles. Existing legislation may need to be modified or removed, or new legislation may be needed to authorize the policy.

In the process of consensus-building, the RAND study suggests that AD stakeholders work together to develop key performance indicators of LTC system performance for persons affected by AD to monitor progressive improvements on each of the five overarching objectives (Shih et al. 2014). Examples include: a target percentage of the estimated population with AD that has received a diagnosis; a target percentage of the Medicaid-eligible diagnosed population that has a quality care plan and is receiving desired home- and community-based services; cross-setting teams and person-centered care plans for a target percentage of persons diagnosed with AD; dementia-specific training received by a target population of caregivers following a diagnosis; and a target percentage reduction in median out-of-pocket LTC costs for persons with AD and their families.

SOCIAL HEALTH AND ALZHEIMER'S

Compared to those without AD, people with AD often are less motivated to engage socially, face more difficulties in organizing activities, are embarrassed by their difficulties in communication, or are worried they might not be able to manage normal activities. Also, social norms and low tolerance for cognitive decline of others can result in their isolation. Even in the early stages of cognitive decline, people report feeling lonelier than people with intact cognition (Cohen-Mansfield et al. 2009). Although family members and friends might initially increase contact after diagnosis, their visits tend to decline as the symptoms become more severe, because they find it too distressing. Moreover, those with more severe AD might be forced to locate away from their previous social support network (Livingston et al. 2017).

Although there is considerable academic and media coverage on how cognitive deficits inhibit independence, less attention has focused on social functioning and the capacity to maintain social relationships (Dröes et al. 2017). Because social relationships have considerable impact on the quality of life of AD patients, it is crucial that the social consequences of dementia receive scrutiny (O'Rourke et al. 2015). According to Huber et al. (2011), social health is characterized by three dimensions: (1) the capacity to fulfill one's potential and obligations; (2) the ability to manage life with some degree of independence, and (3) participation in social activities including work. Dröes et al. (2017) operationalize the first dimension to include the capacity to: exercise choice and autonomy; maintain own identity (personhood); participate and contribute to the community; give and receive support (reciprocity); collaborate with professionals and caregivers; and participate in decision making. When these capacities are in place the person with AD will be able to fulfill her potential and obligations by reciprocating and participating in personal and community life (Innes and Director 2013; Sabat 2001). Factors influencing this dimension of social health are grouped into four categories:

1. personal factors, including mental wellbeing and a sense of coherence, self-efficacy, mastery, resilience, and the capacity to endure stigmatization (Sabat 2001);
2. disease-related factors such as the severity of cognitive disabilities, the diminished learning potential as the disease progresses, and disabilities in performing ADL (Giebel et al. 2015);

3. social factors including the presence or absence of support from a social network; stigma and/or discrimination; the extent to which there is a cooperative relationship with professionals and informal caregivers; and the availability of enriching opportunities; and
4. influencing factors concerning physical and environmental factors in terms of design, living arrangement, the enabling aspect of the environment, and the availability and accessibility of assistive technology.

According to Dröes et al. (2017), there are numerous interventions that can optimize the capability of people with AD to meet their potential and obligations. On a micro level these include building capacities, use of assistive technologies related to social inclusion, and advance care planning while on a macro level they include social inclusion, dementia-friendly communities, and community engagement. The use of assistive technologies (see below) to compensate for functional disabilities regarding memory, orientation, and action can play a role in enabling the patient to function according to their competencies. There are also a set of actions regarding the legal and normative aspects of care to protect and promote the possibility for the AD patient to be part of the decision-making process (Johnson and Karlawish 2015). Basting (2009) emphasizes the importance of activities that focus on the present to improve the lives of persons with AD and offers specific examples of innovative programs that stimulate growth, humor, and emotional connection.

The second dimension, managing life with some degree of independence, involves participation in activities and personal relationships that depend on social factors such as caregiver competence, social support, the living situation (living alone or with a caregiver), and material and environmental factors including the availability of financial resources, dementia-friendly public spaces, and community services such shops, libraries, public transport, and places where social or leisure activities are accessible (Dröes et al. 2017). Shared interventions that have been found effective include self-management group interventions (Toms et al. 2015), home community occupational therapy, and advance care planning interventions (Ampe et al. 2015).

As to the third dimension of social health, the quantity of participation in social activities, such as the number of activities or the size of the social network, alone is not an adequate measure of social health (Kuiper et al. 2015). When evaluating influence of social relationships on AD, it is the quality of participation experienced as meaningful by the person with AD that is critical (Dam et al. 2016). Participation in social activities requires not only the physical ability to attend social activities, but also the cognitive capacity to *actively* share. Often, AD patients feel insecure participating in social activities because of communication difficulties. Moreover, the relative accessibility of the environment, including transport to places where activities are organized, can be a facilitator or barrier to social participation. Overall, strong social networks have a positive impact on physical, mental, and social health and can increase the capacity of communities to involve AD patients and support them emotionally and instrumentally (Wiersma and Denton 2016). Besides connecting them to others, partaking in social activities can provide empowerment, pleasure, and contribute to slowing cognitive deterioration (Kuiper et al. 2015).

There have been a wide variety of test programs designed to facilitate the social health of AD patients. Intergenerational programs involve young adults or children (Park 2014), while other programs include activities with dogs and cats, dolls, singing in chorus, music (King et al. 2018), dance, theater, different types of creative art work and museum visit programs, and even clowns (Kontos et al. 2016). In addition, design guidelines have been developed to increase dementia-friendliness of environments both at home (Gitlin et al. 2009) and in institutional settings (Fleming and Purandare 2010). In Britain, for instance, the concept of dementia-friendly communities is designed to address the social exclusion of AD sufferers by encouraging communities to undertake efforts to provide a high quality of life for those living with AD and enable them to remain living there longer (Innes and Director 2013). They caution, however, that AD patients are heterogeneous which makes care ideals that come in only one size impossible to fit all.

One ambitious innovation, which originated in the Netherlands, is the concept of a dementia village. The first of these was Hogewey, which looks like any village with a theater, restaurants, shops, and apartments surrounding an idyllic courtyard, but is home to 152 men and women with severe dementia. It has 23 living units, each shared by six to eight residents. Around-the-clock care is provided by 240 "villagers" who actually are trained geriatric nurses and carers dressed in street clothes. Even the individuals staffing the various village shops are trained in dementia care (Napoletan 2016). Although some criticize it as a costly, artificial Truman Show, proponents see it as providing the most normal possible environment for AD patients.

METHODS TO ENHANCE SOCIAL HEALTH

Cognitive training has engendered considerable interest and debate in both the academic and commercial sectors (Simons et al. 2016). Cognitive training involves strategies or exercises targeting specific cognitive domains, usually with an adaptive level of difficulty. It encompasses a broad set of interventions, often computer-based, aimed at enhancing problem solving, memory, and speed of processing. The Agency for Healthcare Research and Quality's systematic review found that the intensive Advanced Cognitive Training for Independent and Vital Elderly (ACTIVE) trial, that included specific guidance on how to improve performance on a cognitive task during in-person and small-group training sessions with certified trainers over five to six weeks, as well as two booster sessions, provided moderate improvement at two years, although less over time. According to the NASEM (2017), cognitive training can improve cognitive function in the domain trained, but generally does not lead to significant improvements in performance in other domains. However, limited randomized controlled trial (RCT) evidence suggests that, if well designed, cognitive training can improve long-term cognitive function and maintenance of independence in IADLs.

Cognitive stimulation therapy is the psychological approach with the strongest evidence for improving cognition. It consists of group sessions led by a trained coordinator incorporating social activity, reminiscence, and simple cognitive exercises. Woods et al. (2012), however, found that cognitive stimulation therapy might improve self-reported quality of life but had no significant effect on ADL. It is cost-effective for people with mild to moderate AD and is recommended in the UK by the National Institute of Clinical Excellence. Overall, while clearly efficacious, the evidence that this therapy reaches the threshold for a minimum clinically important difference is debatable, and it might not be effective in all settings (Huntley et al. 2015). Similarly, cognitive rehabilitation aims to improve everyday function by helping the patient set individual goals and devising strategies to achieve these, and might be useful for patients with mild to moderate AD.

Dignity therapy is a short psychotherapeutic intervention that uses a trained therapist to take the person with AD through a guided interview process, producing a "generativity" document that creates a lasting, written legacy during a time when they are still able to communicate

(Johnston et al. 2016). Although meaningful communication becomes more difficult with AD progression, any improvements in communication can have positive effects on the person's dignity and quality of life and can enhance person-centered care. Similarly, shared decision making (SDM) is a means of allowing people with AD to take part in making choices, be autonomous, and participate in social activities (Mariani et al. 2017). Although including families and AD patients in decision making can be challenging for care staff, SDM is an important way of promoting social health. Communication skills training for professionals, training of family caregivers, and involvement of the management in the implementation process are crucial factors in successfully implementing SDM in nursing homes.

Assistive Technologies

Assistive technology may enable persons with AD to remain independent for a longer time, support and assist caregivers and professionals in improving care, and potentially lead to cost savings by delaying entry into care facilities and nursing homes. Meiland et al. (2017) define assistive technology as any item, piece of equipment, product, or system driven by electronics, whether acquired commercially, off-the-shelf, modified, or customized, that is used to help persons with dementia in dealing with its consequences. The technology does not necessarily need to be purposely designed for persons with AD: many technologies can be adapted to their needs. Studies have found that persons with AD are generally positive about using electronic devices to facilitate their independence and reduce family stress (Gitlin et al. 2010). The term "assistive technology," then, includes a wide range of aids, appliances, and system applications in the following areas:

1. Devices intended to help persons living with AD manage their everyday life, such as electronic calendars and medication reminders, aids to perform activities of daily life, robots (Robinson et al. 2013), navigation systems, and safety devices;
2. Technologies to help AD patients engage in satisfying and enjoyable activities such as cognitive stimulation and physical activities, or to improve social participation and contact;
3. Caregiver support technologies to help with the care of the AD patient or improve their own wellbeing;

4. Health care technologies that support professional organizations and systems within AD health and social care, such as behavior monitoring and Global Positioning System tracking systems.

Despite the potential benefits of technological support systems, several impediments remain before they will make a genuine difference in AD care. These include their prevailing use for safety and security rather than for lifestyle in general, their slow uptake and implementation, the scarcity of quality scientific research as to their efficacy and cost-effectiveness for AD care (Fleming and Sum 2014), and a lack of concern to aesthetics which can make them seem stigmatizing (Knapp et al. 2015). Furthermore, to develop usable technological solutions, it is crucial to understand how persons with AD can access and embrace the technology. Unless a good match between the person and the technology is achieved from the user's perspective, the technology may be ignored or not used optimally (Meiland et al. 2017). Little things count; for instance, research on the preferences of persons with AD confirms that touchscreen devices are preferred over mouse or keyboard devices because they reduce the distance between the user and the result, thus enhancing his or her involvement in the task (Meiland, et al. 2017). Importantly, given the progressive nature of AD, the patient's acceptance of and ability to use assistive technologies will diminish over their course (Hedman et al. 2015). Therefore, certain devices might have a window of usefulness and timing is of the essence (Livingston et al. 2017; Burstein et al. 2014).

Many devices have been tested within the domain of technologies for meaningful or pleasurable activities. For example, sensors and smart home technologies provide a valuable visual of performed activities and reportedly are successful in preventing major incidents. Woolham (2005) concluded that smart home technologies help persons with AD by improving confidence, extending home and community living, and reducing the need for care visits. Moreover, use of assistive technologies is expected to expand with the increase in computer literacy and education levels of future generations of older people. The aim of technological innovations should be to improve care without unreasonably increasing risks for people with AD and their families, thus preserving privacy and autonomy for the patient is crucial. While some devices have the potential to enhance safety, they raise concerns of replacing or reducing human contact (Connelly et al. 2014). For Livingston et al. (2017), technology should never be a replacement for human contact. Also, the development and use of devices used to restrict or restrain people with AD raise special concerns. To date, there has been little research regarding the potential of social media to increase access to social support and interaction for people with AD or how religiosity/spirituality plays a role in fulfilling one's potential and affects the experience of personhood.

SUMMARY

In the absence of innovative policy initiatives, LTC will become a progressively more difficult problem facing developed countries first and then LMICs. The shrinking supply of informal caregivers, combined with pressures toward minimum wage scales for a more professional formal care workforce, will escalate the cost of LTC considerably. Moreover, although enhancing the social health of AD patients is a worthy endeavor, it is bound to be an expensive one as well. Overall, then, efforts to rein in the costs of AD will face an uphill battle. One strategy that is receiving growing attention is that of strengthening the public health component of AD and vastly increasing research on preventive measures to, hopefully, reduce the burden in the future. Chapter 5 reviews recent work in health promotion and prevention policy.

REFERENCES

Alper, J. (2006) *The Partnership for Long-term Care: A Public-Private Partnership to Finance Long-term Care.* Robert Wood Johnson Foundation.

Alzheimer's Association (2016) "Alzheimer's disease facts and figures." *Alzheimer's and Dementia* 12 (4). https://www.alz.org/documents_custom/2016-facts-and-figures.pdf.

Alzheimer's Association (2018) "Alzheimer's disease facts and figures." *Alzheimer's and Dementia* 14 (3): 367–429.

Ampe, S., A. Sevenants, E. Coppens, N. Spruytte et al. (2015) "Study protocol for 'we DECide': Implementation of advance care planning for nursing home residents with dementia. *Journal of Advanced Nursing* 71 (5): 1156–62.

Ausserhofer, D., M. Deschodt and S. De Geest (2016) "There's no place like home: A scoping review on the impact of homelike residential care models on resident-, family-, and staff-related outcomes." *Journal of American Medical Directors Association* 17: 685–93.

Ballard, C.A., M. Orrell, S. YongZhong, E. Moniz-Cook et al. (2016) "Impact of antipsychotic review and nonpharmacological intervention on antipsychotic use, neuropsychiatric symptoms, and mortality in people with dementia living in nursing homes: A factorial cluster randomized controlled trial by the Well-Being and Health for People with Dementia (WHELD) program." *American Journal of Psychiatry* 173: 252–62.

Basting, A.D. (2009) *Forget Memory: Creating Better Lives for People with Dementia*. Boston: Johns Hopkins Press.

Beerens, H.C., S.M. Zwakhalen, H. Verbeek, D. Ruwaard and J.P. Hamers (2013) "Factors associated with quality of life of people with dementia in long-term care facilities: A systematic review." *International Journal of Nursing Studies* 50: 1259–70.

Burau, V., H. Theobald and R.H. Blank (2007) *Governing Home Care: A Cross-National Comparison*. London: Edward Elgar.

Burstein, A.A., O. DaDalt, B. Kramer, L. D'Ambrosio and J. Coughlin (2014) "Technology and the caregiving dilemma: A comparative look at awareness, attitudes, and the role of technology." *Alzheimer's and Dementia* 10 (Suppl): 571.

Campbell, J., N. Ikegami, C. Gori, F. Barbabella et al. (2016) "How different countries allocate long-term care resources to older users: A comparative snapshot." In C. Gori, J-L. Fernández and R. Wittenberg, eds., *Long-term Care Reforms in OECD Countries: Successes and Failures*. Bristol: Policy Press, pp. 47–76.

Cohen-Mansfield, J., D. Shmotkin and S. Goldberg (2009) "Loneliness in old age: Longitudinal changes and their determinants in an Israeli sample." *International Journal of Psychogeriatrics* 21: 1160–70

Commission on Long-Term Care (2013) *A Comprehensive Approach to Long-Term Services and Supports*. Washington, DC: Commission on Long-Term Care

Connelly, K., K. ur Rehman Laghari, M. Mokhtari and T.H. Falk (2014) "Approaches to understanding the impact of technologies for aging in place: A mini-review." *Gerontology* 60: 282–88

Cooper, C., A. Selwood, M. Blanchard, Z. Walker et al. (2010) "The determinants of family carers' abusive behaviour to people with dementia: Results of the CARD study." *Journal of Affective Disorders* 121: 136–42

Corbett, A., J. Stevens, D. Aarsland et al. (2012) "Systematic review of services providing information and/or advice to people with dementia and/or their caregivers." *International Journal of Geriatric Psychiatry* 27: 628–36

Dam, A.E., M.E. de Vugt, I.P. Klinkenberg, F.R. Verhey, and M.P. van Boxtel (2016) "A systematic review of social support interventions for caregivers of people with dementia: Are they doing what they promise?" *Maturitas* 85: 117–30.

Department of Health and Human Services (DHHS) (2014) National Alzheimer's Project Act. http://aspe.hhs.gov/daltcp/napa/.

Dong X., R. Chen and M.A. Simon (2014) "Elder abuse and dementia: A review of the research and health policy." *Health Affairs* 33 (4): 642–49.

Doty, P. (2010) "The evolving balance of formal and informal, institutional and non-institutional long-term care for older Americans: A thirty-year perspective." *Public Policy and Aging Report* 20 (1): 3–9.

Dröes, R.M., R. Chattat, A. Diaz, D. Gove et al. (2017) "Social health and dementia: A European consensus on the operationalization of the concept and directions for research and practice." *Aging and Mental Health* 21 (1): 4–17.

Eisenberg, R. (2017) "The troubling AARP long-term care scorecard." *Forbes.* https://www.forbes.com/sites/nextavenue/2017/06/14/the-troubling-aarp-long-term-care-scorecard/#2c7fccde6b25.

Feinberg, L., S.C. Reinhard, A. Houser and R. Choula (2011) *Valuing the Invaluable: 2011 Update: The Growing Contributions and Costs of Family Caregiving.* Washington, DC: AARP Public Policy Institute.

Fleming, R. and N. Purandare (2010) "Long-term care for people with dementia: Environmental design guidelines." *International Psychogeriatrics* 22 (7): 1084–96.

Fleming, R. and S. Sum (2014) "Empirical studies on the effectiveness of assistive technology in the care of people with dementia: A systematic review." *Journal of Assistive Technologies* 8 (1): 14–34.

Gallagher, D., A. Ni Mhaolain, L. Crosby et al. (2013) "Determinants of the desire to institutionalize in Alzheimer's caregivers." *American Journal of Alzheimer's Disease and Other Dementias* 26: 205–11.

Giebel, C.M., D. Challisand and D. Montaldi (2015) "Understanding the cognitive underpinnings of functional impairments in early dementia: A review." *Aging and Mental Health* 19 (10): 859–75.

Gitlin, L.N., L. Winter and M. Dennis (2010) "Assistive devices caregivers use and find helpful to manage problem behaviors of dementia." *Gerontechnology* 9 (3): 408–14.

Gitlin, L.N., W.W. Hauck, M.P. Dennis, L. Winter et al. (2009) "Long-term effect on mortality of a home intervention that reduces functional difficulties in older adults: Results from a randomized trial." *Journal of the American Geriatrics Society* 57 (3): 476–81.

Goren, A., W. Montgomery, K. Kahle-Wrobleski, T. Nakamura and K. Ueda (2016) "Impact of caring for persons with Alzheimer's disease or dementia on caregivers' health outcomes: Findings from a community based survey in Japan." *BMC Geriatrics* 16: 122.

Hedman, A., L. Nygård, O. Almkvist and A. Kottorp (2015) "Amount and type of everyday technology use over time in older adults with cognitive impairment." *Scandinavian Journal of Occupational Therapy* 22 (3): 196–206.

Houser, A., M.J. Gibson and D. Redfoot (2010) "Trends in family caregiving and paid home care for older people with disabilities in the community." Washington, DC: AARP Public Policy Institute.

Huber, M., J.A. Knottnerus, L. Green and H. van der Horst (2011) "How should we define health?" *British Medical Journal* 343: d4163.

Huntley, J.D., R.L. Gould, K. Liu, M. Smith and R.J. Howard (2015) "Do cognitive interventions improve general cognition in dementia? A meta-analysis and meta-regression." *BMJ Open* 5: e005247.

Innes, A. and B. Director (2013) "Working towards dementia friendly societies." *Perspectives in Public Health* 133 (3): 141.

Johnson, R.A. and J. Karlawish (2015) "A review of ethical issues in dementia." *International Psychogeriatric* 27 (10): 1635–47.

Johnston, B., S. Lawton, C. McCaw, E. Law et al. (2016) "Living well with dementia: Enhancing dignity and quality of life, using a novel intervention, dignity therapy." *International Journal of Older People Nursing* 11 (2): 107–20.

Keenan, T.A. (2010) "Planning for long-term care: A survey of midlife and older women." AARP Research Report.

King, J.B., K.G. Jones, E. Goldberg, M. Rollins, K. MacNamee et al. (2018) "Increased functional connectivity after listening to favoured music in adults with Alzheimer dementia." *The Journal of Prevention of Alzheimer's Disease.* https://doi.org/10.14283/jpad.2018.19.

Knapp, M., J. Barlow, A. Comras-Herrera et al. (2015) "The case for investment in technology to manage the global costs of dementia." http://eprints.lse.ac.uk/66482/1/__lse.ac.uk_storage_LIBRARY_Secondary_libfile_shared_repository_Content_LSEE_The%20case%20for%20investment%20in%20technology.

Koivisto, A.M., I. Hallikainen, T. Välimäki et al. (2016) "Early psychosocial intervention does not delay institutionalization in persons with mild Alzheimer disease and has impact on neither disease progression nor caregivers' well-being: ALSOVA 3-year follow-up." *International Journal of Geriatric Psychiatry* 31: 273–83.

Kontos, P., K.L. Miller, R. Colobong, L.I. Palma Lazgare et al. (2016) "Elder-clowning in long-term dementia care: Results of a pilot study." *Journal of the American Geriatrics Society* 64 (2): 347–53.

Kuiper, J.S., M. Zuidersma, R.C. Oude Voshaar, S.U. Zuidema et al. (2015) "Social relationships and risk of dementia: A systematic review and meta-analysis of longitudinal cohort studies." *Ageing Research Reviews* 22: 39–57.

Lai, C.K., J.H. Yeung, V. Mok and I. Chi (2009) "Special care units for dementia individuals with behavioural problems." *Cochrane Database Systems Review* 4: CD006470.

Livingston, G., J. Barber, P. Rapaport et al. (2014) "START (STrAtegies for RelaTives) study: A pragmatic randomised controlled trial to determine the clinical effectiveness and cost-effectiveness of a manual-based coping strategy programme in promoting the mental health of carers of people with dementia." *Health Technology Assessment* 18: 1–242.

Livingston, G., A. Sommerlad, V. Orgeta, S.G. Costafreda et al. (2017) "Dementia prevention, intervention, and care." *The Lancet.* https://doi.org/10.1016/S0140-6736(17)31363-6.

Mariani, E., M. Vernooij-Dassen, R. Koopmans, Y. Engels and R. Chattat (2017) "Shared decision-making in dementia care planning: Barriers and facilitators in two European countries." *Aging & Mental Health* 21 (1): 31–39.

Meiland, F., A. Innes, G. Mountain, L. Robinson, et al. (2017) "Technologies to support community-dwelling persons with dementia: A position paper on issues regarding development, usability, effectiveness and cost-effectiveness, deployment, and ethics." *JMIR Rehabilitation and Assistive Technologies* 4 (1): e1. https://doi.org/10.2196/rehab.6376.

MetLife Mature Market Institute (2010) *The MetLife Study of Working Caregivers and Employer Health Care Costs.* Westport, CT: MetLife Mature Market Institute.

MetLife Mature Market Institute (2011) *The MetLife Study of Caregiving Costs to Working Caregivers: Double Jeopardy for Baby Boomers Caring for Their Parents.* Westport, CT: MetLife Mature Market Institute.

Moyle, W. and S. O'Dwyer (2012) "Quality of life in people living with dementia in nursing homes." *Current Opinions in Psychiatry* 25: 480–84.

Nadash, P. and Y-C. Shih (2012) "Introducing social insurance for long-term care in Taiwan: Key issues." *International Journal of Social Welfare.* https://doi.org/10.1111/j.1468-2397.2011.00862.x.

Napoletan, A. (2016) "Dementia care: What in the world is a dementia village?" http://www.alzheimers.net/2013-08-07/dementia-village/.

National Academies of Sciences, Engineering, and Medicine (NASEM) (2017) *Preventing Cognitive Decline and Dementia: A Way Forward.* Washington, DC: The National Academies Press.

National Association of State Units on Aging (2005) *Nursing Home Abuse Risk Prevention Profile and Checklist.* Washington, DC: National Center on Elder Abuse.

Naylor, M.D., L.H. Aiken, E.T. Kurtzman, D.M. Olds and K.B. Hirshman (2011) "The importance of transitional care in achieving health reform." *Health Affairs* 30 (4): 746–54.

Ng, T., C. Harrington, M. Musumeci and E.L. Reaves (2014) *Medicaid Home and Community-Based Services Programs: 2010 Data Update.* Washington, DC: Kaiser Family Foundation.

O'Rourke, H.M., W. Duggleby, K.D. Fraser and L. Jerke (2015) "Factors that affect quality of life from the perspective of people with dementia: A metasynthesis." *Journal of the American Geriatrics Society* 63 (1): 24–38.

Park, A-L. (2014) "Is there anything special about intergenerational approaches to older people with dementia? A review." *Journal of Alzheimer's Disease & Parkinsonism* 4: 172–80.

Pavolini, E. and H. Theobald (2015) "Long-term care policies." In E. Kuhlmann, R.H. Blank, I.L. Bourgeault and C. Wendt, eds., *The Palgrave International Handbook of Healthcare Policy and Governance.* Basingstoke: Palgrave, pp. 462–78.

Ramnarace, C. (2010) "The high costs of caring for Alzheimer's patients." http://www.aarp.org/relationships/caregiving/info-10-2010/the_high_costs_of_caring_for_alzheimers_patients.html.

Rapaport, P., G. Livingston, A. Mulla, J. Murray and C. Cooper (2017) "A systematic review of the effective components of psychosocial interventions delivered by care home staff to people with dementia." *BMJ Open* 7: e014177.

Redfoot, D., L. Feinberg and A. Houser (2013) *The Aging of the Baby Boom and the Growing Care Gap: A Look at Future Declines in the Availability of Family Caregivers.* Washington, DC: AARP Public Policy Institute.

Reinhard, S.C., E. Kassner, A. Houser, K. Ujvari et al. (2014) "Raising expectations: A state scorecard on long-term services and supports for older adults, people with physical disabilities, and family caregivers." http://www.longtermscorecard.org/.

Robinson, H., B. Macdonald, N. Kerse and E. Broadbent (2013) "The psychosocial effects of a companion robot: A randomized controlled trial." *Journal of the American Medical Directors Association* 14: 661–67.

Sabat, S.R. (2001) *The Experience of Alzheimer's Disease: Life Through a Tangled Veil.* Oxford, UK: Blackwell Publishers.

SCAN Foundation (2013) "Who pays for long-term care in the U.S.?" Long Beach, CA: SCAN Foundation. http://www.thescanfoundation.org/who-pays-long-term-care-us.

Schubert, C.C., M. Callahan, C.M. Perkins, A.J. Hui and H.C. Hendrie (2008) "Acute care utilization by dementia caregivers within urban primary care practices." *Journal of General Internal Medicine* 23 (11): 1736–40.

Shih, R.A., T.W. Concannon, J.L. Liu and E.M. Friedman (2014) "Improving dementia long-term care: A policy blueprint." *Rand Health Quarterly* 4 (2): 2.

Simons, D.J., W.R. Boot, N. Charness, S.E. Gathercole et al. (2016) "Do "brain-training" programs work?" *Psychological Science in the Public Interest* 17 (3): 103–86.

Smith, M., K.C. Buckwalter, H. Kang, V. Ellingrod and S.K. Schultz (2008) "Dementia-specific assisted living: Clinical factors and psychotropic medication use." *Journal of the American Psychiatric Nurses Association* 14: 39–49.

Spillman, B.C. and S.K. Long (2009) "Does high caregiver stress predict nursing home entry?" *Inquiry* 46: 140–61.

Theobald, H. and S. Hampel (2013) "Radical institutional change and incremental transformation: Long-term care insurance in Germany." In C. Ranci and E. Pavolini, eds., *Reforms in Long-term Care Policies in Europe.* Heidelberg and New York: Springer, pp. 117–38.

Theobald, H. and E. Ozanne (2016) "Multi-level governance and its effects in long-term care policies." In C. Gori, J-L. Fernández and R. Wittenberg, eds., *Long-term Care Reforms in OECD Countries: Successes and Failures.* Bristol: Policy Press, pp. 271–92.

Toms, G.R., C. Quinn, D.E. Anderson and L. Clare (2015) "Help yourself per-spectives on self-management from people with dementia and their caregivers." *Qualitative Health Research* 25 (1): 87–98.

Verbeek, H., E. van Rossum, S.M. Zwakhalen, G.I. Kempen and J.P. Hamers (2009) "Small, homelike care environments for older people with dementia: A literature review." *International Psychogeriatrics* 21: 252–64.

Wakabayashi, C. and K.M. Donato (2006) "Does caregiving increase poverty among women in later life? Evidence from the Health and Retirement Survey." *Journal of Health and Social Behavior* 47 (3): 258–74.

Wiersma, E.C. and A. Denton (2016) "From social network to safety net: Dementia-friendly communities in rural Northern Ontario." *Dementia* 15 (1): 51–68.

Wolff, J. L., J. Feder and R. Schulz (2016) "Supporting family caregivers of older Americans." *New England Journal of Medicine* 375 (26): 2513–15.

Woods, B., E. Aguirre, A.E. Spector and M. Orrell (2012) "Cognitive stimulation to improve cognitive functioning in people with dementia." *Cochrane Database System Review* 2: CD005562.

Woolham, J. (2005) *Safe at Home: The Effectiveness of Assistive Technology in Supporting the Independence of People with Dementia: The Safe at Home Project.* London: Hawker Press.

Zimmerman, S., W.L. Anderson, S. Brode et al. (2013) "Systematic review: Effective characteristics of nursing homes and other residential long-term care settings for people with dementia." *Journal of the American Geriatrics Society* 61: 1399–409.

CHAPTER 5

Public Health Approaches to Alzheimer's Disease

Abstract Shifts in disease burdens toward chronic long-term conditions like AD, along with the high costs of acute care in aging populations, have led to a renaissance of interest in health promotion and preventive policies in many countries. This chapter summarizes the latest evidence of potential risk-reduction and prevention strategies that cumulatively might prevent up to one-third of AD cases in the future. It examines this evidence across a wide array of potential interventions, some of which have proven to be inauspicious to date. If the goal of the health care system is to improve the health of the population, public health programs, particularly those that produce healthier lifestyles, are critical.

Keywords Disease burden • Preventative policies • Public health programs

Despite convincing evidence that the most significant advances in the health of populations have come from outside medicine, many forces, particularly the medical professions and the health care industry, have strong economic interests in maintaining or increasing acute care. In combination with patients, and a public easily swayed by optimistic media coverage, they have aggrandized curative medicine at the expense of public health. If the goal of the health care system is to improve the health of the

R. H. Blank, *Social & Public Policy of Alzheimer's Disease in the United States*, https://doi.org/10.1007/978-981-13-0656-3_5

population, however, public health programs, particularly those that produce healthier lifestyles, are critical. Despite these strong forces behind a medical model, shifts in disease burdens toward chronic long-term conditions like AD, along with the high costs of acute care in aging populations, have led to a renaissance of interest in health promotion and preventive policies in many countries.

Emerging Public Health Initiatives for AD

According to former Surgeon General David Sacher, "Alzheimer's is the most under-recognized threat to public health in the 21st century" (Alzheimer's Impact Movement 2018). In response, in April 2018 a bipartisan bill, Building Our Largest Dementia (BOLD) Infrastructure for Alzheimer's Act (S. 2076/H.R. 4256), was introduced in Congress. If enacted, the bill would create an AD public health infrastructure across the United States to implement effective AD interventions focused on public health issues such as increasing early detection and diagnosis, reducing risk, and preventing avoidable hospitalizations. It would also increase implementation of the Healthy Brain Initiative's *Public Health Road Map* nationwide by establishing Alzheimer's centers of excellence, providing cooperative agreements to public health departments, and increasing data collection, analysis, and timely reporting (Alzheimer's Impact Movement 2018).

Concurrently, AD has become a public health priority worldwide through the efforts of organizations, such as Alzheimer Europe and Alzheimer Disease International (Innes and Director 2013). The first item of the Paris Declaration, which lists the political priorities of the European Alzheimer movement, is the call for national governments to recognize AD as a major public health challenge and develop national action programs. This was supported by the recommendation of Alzheimer Europe that governments devise national action plans for AD care and provide the funds necessary to implement them (for a useful summary of the status of existing and developing national dementia strategies in Europe, see Alzheimer Europe 2016).

On May 29, 2017, the World Health Assembly endorsed the WHO Global Action Plan on the Public Health Response to Dementia (2017–2025) (WHO 2017) with member states committing to international collaboration and national strategies with implementation plans.

The Global Plan aims to improve the lives of people with AD and their caregivers and to decrease its burden on communities and countries. Its multiple priorities include: reducing the risk of dementia; diagnosis, treatment, and care; research and innovative technologies; and development of supportive environments for carers. This plan signals an upswing in awareness of the need to address what WHO declared, in 2012, to be a global public health priority. However, concerted international and intersectoral collaborative action, which to date has been wanting, will be required to implement WHO's Plan.

The modest target in the WHO Global Action Plan is that half of all countries will have diagnosed half of all AD cases by 2025. An important part of the solution is to move to task-sharing models in which most care is delivered by non-specialist primary care and community services (Prince 2017). In LMICs there are too few specialists to provide services for more than a small proportion of AD patients. Primary care staff are well situated to deliver care that is holistic, integrated, and person-centered in LMICs as well as HICs. According to the Lancet Commission, there is much potential for South–North learning and knowledge transfer. HICs do not have a monopoly on solutions, and, it could be argued, have developed a poorly integrated, overspecialized model of care that fails to meet the needs of many AD patients (Prince 2017).

These international efforts have resulted in a policy context that drives agendas supporting earlier diagnosis, improvements in post-diagnostic support, and better standards of care in hospitals, care homes, and the community. For instance, in Britain the Prime Minister's Challenge on Dementia has set clear expectations that more funding should be dedicated not only to research seeking to find evidence on how to better support people with AD, but also to improve current care practices and emphasize preventive strategies. Recommendations from the Productivity Commission and Dementia Australia, the Government Office for Science in the UK, and the Presidential Commission for the Study of Bioethical Issues and the IOM in the United States, among others, encourage older adults to engage in mental, physical, and social activities for healthy cognitive aging. While Forlini and Hall (2017) agree that these efforts are timely, they warn that ethical tensions arise when this individual responsibility collides with social and personal realities of aging populations.

Reducing the Risk of AD and Promoting Cognitive Health

In part a result of these initiatives, more attention has begun to concentrate on the expectation that brain health promotion and risk reduction could eventually moderate the impact of the AD epidemic (Norton et al. 2014). Although caution is warranted, the message that some AD might be preventable through effective implementation of public health strategies is one that policy makers and public need to hear and act on (Prince 2017). According to the Lancet Commission on Dementia Prevention and Care (Livingston et al. 2017), AD is by no means an inevitable consequence of aging. Lifestyle factors might reduce, or increase, an individual's risk of developing it. Some AD risk factors, including cardiovascular and cerebrovascular disease, metabolic and psychiatric factors, diet, lifestyle, and education, are potentially modifiable (Norton et al. 2014). By incorporating potentially reversible risk factors from different phases of the life span and not just old age, the Commission calculated that, theoretically, more than a third of AD cases might be preventable. An increase in childhood education and exercise, maintenance of social contacts, smoking abatement, as well as management of hearing loss, depression, diabetes, hypertension, and obesity could all contribute to prevention or delay of AD (Livingston et al. 2017). Although not everyone will be able to make necessary changes and some changes will not make a difference (and some risks of AD are genetic and not currently modifiable), delaying AD for a few years for even a small percentage of the population could be an enormous achievement and enable more to live their life without developing it.

The Lancet Commission based many of its prevention inferences on the theory of cognitive reserve or resilience. As noted earlier, it has long been recognized that some people with neuropathological changes of AD do not develop dementia (Cholerton et al. 2013). This has led to the concept of cognitive reserve, that people who have such brain reserve can tolerate more neuropathology without cognitive and functional decline and will develop AD more slowly than people without this type of brain reserve. Thus, cognitive resilience in later life is enhanced by building brain reserve earlier in life through education and other intellectual stimulation (Borenstein and Mortimer 2016). Not surprisingly, higher educational achievement in early life has consistently been associated with reduced risk of AD (Satizabal et al. 2016; Meng and D'Arcy 2012).

Although the scientific evidence on how to prevent or delay cognitive deterioration has been limited at best, and despite the many exaggerated claims made in popular media and the marketing of products raised in Chap. 3, a growing body of prevention research is emerging. The first systematic review published in 2010 by the Agency for Healthcare Research and Quality (AHRQ) and an associated conference at the NIH concluded that there was insufficient evidence to make recommendations about interventions to prevent cognitive decline and AD. Since then, understanding of the pathological processes that result in AD has advanced significantly, and many clinical trials of potential preventive interventions have been published. During the 2016 G7 summit in Japan, an array of national science academies highlighted global brain research as a critical priority, including a call for global programs on diagnosing, preventing, and treating brain disorders such as AD (G-Science Academies 2016). Similarly, the WHO's *Global Action Plan on the Public Health Response to Dementia 2017–2025* includes prevention as an important action area (WHO 2017a). Likewise, the Alzheimer's Association recently examined the evidence on modifiable risk factors for cognitive decline and AD (Baumgart et al. 2015) while a 2015 Institute of Medicine (IOM) report took an in-depth look at the evidence on cognitive aging (IOM 2015). Furthermore, AARP launched a Global Council on Brain Health to bring together scientists, health professionals, and others to develop evidence-based recommendations on lifestyle changes that may impact brain health (AARP 2017).

A fundamental question is when in the life span should AD prevention programs be implemented and for how long. Mounting evidence from epidemiological, clinical, imaging, and biomarker studies suggests that AD is a clinically silent disorder beginning decades earlier, whose terminal phase is characterized by dementia (Frankish and Horton 2017). In other words, although AD is usually diagnosed later in life, the pathology develops years, or even decades, earlier, thus any preventive measures must begin early in life (Ritchie et al. 2015).

The Lancet Neurology Commission suggests that the goal of interventions that affect the long-term course of AD should not only slow disease progression, but also minimize the time with severe AD and maximize the time with preserved cognitive resources, autonomy, and quality of life (Winblad et al. 2016). If late-stage morbidity is compressed and patients spend proportionally more time in less severe states, cost savings could be substantial. If, on the other hand, interventions improve survival, but prolong the time with severe AD, they might bring about some marginal health benefits for patients but would increase care costs and burdens substantially. Therefore, to delay the onset of AD, the optimum time for interventions that target lifestyle-related cardiovascular and risk factors is most likely young adulthood or middle age, with interventions that target multiple domains more likely to be effective. Evidence, therefore, must be assessed from a life-course perspective (Winblad et al. 2016).

The NASEM's Report *Preventing Cognitive Decline and Dementia: A Way Forward* (2017) examines the current evidence of interventions for preventing cognitive decline and AD. The report incorporates the 2017 AHRQ systematic review to summarize the state of evidence on the effectiveness and harms of interventions associated with preventing or delaying the onset or slowing the progression of CATD, MCI, and AD. It takes a more cautious approach than the Lancet Commissions and other panels by focusing primarily on available evidence from randomized controlled trials (RCTs) and only secondarily on observational non-experimental studies and evidence from studies of risk factors and neurobiological studies. The AHRQ study found only modest RCT evidence for only a few classes of interventions (Kane et al. 2017). Overall, the Committee determined that evidence remains relatively restricted and bears significant shortcomings that stem, in part, from the difficulties inherent in conducting RCTs on interventions for conditions with long latency periods that are often comorbid with other late-life conditions. Nevertheless, they recommend that, when communicating with the public, the NIH and other public health organizations should make clear the potential positive effects of intensive cognitive training, blood pressure management, and increased physical activity. Before investing in public health strategies that strongly advance the adoption of these interventions, however, additional research is needed to better understand and gain confidence in their effectiveness.

Population-based estimates of the percentage of AD cases attributable to each factor by the Lancet Commission suggest that nine potentially modifiable risk factors may account for 35 percent of AD cases in the United States and Europe (Livingston et al. 2017). Even a modest 10 percent reduction in each of these risk factors could reduce the prevalence of AD by about 8 percent by 2050 (Norton et al. 2014). Thus, public health strategies targeting these lifestyle, clinical, and social risk factors could reduce the incidence of AD or delay its onset. Naturally, prevention of all potentially modifiable cases of AD is not feasible, but even pushing back the age of onset slightly could bring enormous benefits. Estimates suggest that a delay in onset of one year could prevent more than nine million cases of dementia by 2050 and delaying onset by five years could halve the prevalence of dementia globally (Frankish and Horton 2017). Undoubtedly, multi-modal mediations would be necessary to prevent progression from MCI to AD. These interventions might involve approaches to reduce neuropathological damage (treating vascular risk factors, diabetes, diet, exercise), combined with those that maximize function (cognitive and social stimulation, treatment of neuropsychiatric symptoms). Understanding which components are most worthwhile and how to simplify and make them cost-efficient is critical (Livingston et al. 2017).

It is important to caution that increased longevity and the baby boom generation mean that the overall number of people with AD will still increase markedly in the coming decades even with prevention efforts (Larson and Langa 2017). Furthermore, its burden will be felt most acutely among minorities (Mayeda et al. 2014) and economically disadvantaged populations (Yaffe et al. 2013), as well as among the oldest old. Ironically, reduction of risk exposures is likely to lower incidence but increase survival, with a neutral effect on age-specific AD prevalence (Prince et al. 2016). For example, cardiovascular health is deteriorating in many LMICs and even with preventive action, AD incidence in these settings could increase (Moll van Charante et al. 2016). Therefore, Frankish and Horton (2017) call on all governments to generate updated action plans for AD, drawing on the latest evidence and incorporating awareness strategies and public health campaigns, to confront the impending AD crisis. Prevention will not solve the problem, but it might make it more manageable and, in the process, help many individuals avoid the ravages of AD.

Although there is growing evidence that certain preventive strategies might be effective, many of the purported approaches promoted to that end (discussed in Chap. 3) are not viable candidates. The following areas have the most potential based on the provisional evidence collected to date.

Increased Education

There is persuasive evidence that people with little formal education are at an increased risk of developing AD (Larson et al. 2013). As noted above, the theory is that education enriches the cognitive reserve, making one's brain less vulnerable to cognitive decline. Conversely, low educational levels result in vulnerability to cognitive decline because the brain has less reserve to help maintain cognitive function (Livingston et al. 2017). In the Framingham Heart Study, for example, a decline in AD incidence was found for those participants with at least a high school diploma (Satizabal et al. 2016). According to the NASEM (2017), however, education is an indicator of socioeconomic status, making it difficult to disentangle the effects of each. Variation in risk by socioeconomic status also was demonstrated by Yaffe et al. (2013) who found that variation in AD risk between white and black participants was no longer statistically significant after controlling for socioeconomic status. Globally, the Lancet Commission estimates that global AD cases could be reduced by 8 percent if all people continued their education until at least age 15. In later life, continuing education might enhance cognitive reserve, although the evidence is limited at present.

Blood Pressure Management

Numerous links exist between cerebrovascular disease and AD. Most AD patients show evidence of it, often in combination with Alzheimer's pathology (Rahimi and Kovacs 2014). Epidemiologic data also demonstrate that both clinical stroke and subclinical cerebrovascular disease are important risk factors for AD. It is plausible that blood pressure management, including medications and lifestyle-based strategies, such as diet, weight control, and exercise, for people with hypertension could reduce the risk of cognitive decline and AD. Managing blood pressure, particularly during midlife, to prevent, delay, or slow the progression of AD is supported by promising, though inconclusive, evidence. This, together with the strong support for blood pressure management in preventing stroke and cardiovascular disease and the relative benefit/risk ratio of antihypertensive medications and lifestyle interventions, is sufficient to justify informing the public about the use of blood pressure management as a preventive strategy (NASEM 2017).

Physical Activity

It is also well documented that physical activity has many health benefits and that some of these benefits are causally related to brain health. An IOM report concludes that increased exercise in midlife is associated with a reduced risk of AD (IOM 2015). While exercise alone does not appear to improve cognition in healthy older adults (Young et al. 2015), those who do so regularly are more likely to maintain cognition than those who are sedentary. Results of one meta-analysis reported that physical activity had a significant protective effect against cognitive decline, with high levels of exercise being the most protective (Sofi et al. 2011). The NASEM report recommends exercise to delay or slow age-related cognitive decline, and other studies suggest that tai chi, longer exercise sessions, and resistance training may all have particular benefits for the brain. ten Brinke et al. (2017) found that aerobic training significantly improved left, right, and total hippocampal volume while Chirles et al. (2017) found even moderately intense walking increased connectivity in ten brain regions spanning the frontal, parietal, temporal, and insular lobes and the cerebellum, thus demonstrating the protective effects of exercise training on the cognitive reserve.

A large 44-year study of Swedish women found that a high cardiovascular fitness in midlife was associated with a decreased risk of dementia. According to the authors, promotion of a high cardiovascular fitness should be included in strategies to mitigate or prevent dementia (Hörder et al. 2018). In their meta-analysis of 19 studies that examined the effect of exercise training programs on cognitive function in older adults who were at risk for or diagnosed with AD, Panza et al. (2018) concluded that those who exercised showed small improvements in cognitive function no matter what type of exercise they did, whereas older adults in the no-exercise control groups faced declines in cognitive function.

Importantly, individuals can change their behavior to increase physical activity at any age and doing so does not necessarily require adherence to a structured exercise program. Moreover, physical activity levels can be boosted by work or leisure activities and be influenced by community conditions such as the availability of neighborhood green space or bike paths (Dalton et al. 2016). Barnes and Yaffe (2011) estimate that nearly 4.3 million AD cases globally and over one million cases in the United States could be attributed to physical inactivity, and a 25 percent reduction could potentially prevent nearly one million cases globally and 230,000 in the United States.

Smoking

The link between smoking and AD could be related to the many ill effects smoking has on cardiovascular health, but cigarette smoke also contains substances that are toxic to the brain, further compounding the risk. The

Lancet Commission estimates the number of AD cases worldwide could be reduced by 5 percent if all people stopped smoking. It is particularly important to stop smoking later in life to reduce neurotoxins and improve heart, lung, and brain health.

Weight Control

Obesity is a key risk factor in middle age, especially for those who develop a hormonal condition called insulin resistance. But the relationship between weight and AD risk is complex as evidenced by a study of nearly two million people in Britain which found that being underweight in midlife was also associated with an increased risk of AD (Qizilbash et al. 2015). Compared with people of a healthy weight, underweight people had a 34 percent higher risk of AD. Furthermore, the incidence of AD continued to fall for every increasing body mass index (BMI) category, with very obese people having a 29 percent lower AD risk than people of a healthy weight.

Depression

While there are definite links between depression and AD, there is debate as to the direction of causation: is depression a prodromal symptom of AD or an independent risk factor for AD? According to the Lancet researchers, depression in later life may make people more vulnerable to AD because it increases stress hormone levels and adversely affects the growth and survival of neuronal growth factors and hippocampal volume.

Social Engagement

A growing body of evidence from observational and intervention studies on the cognitive benefits of participation in social activities suggests that engaging in social activities may help prevent cognitive decline and AD (IOM 2015). Loneliness and a lack of physical contact, especially later in life, are linked to a constellation of health problems, including heart disease, hypertension, and depression. Social isolation is tied to cognitive inactivity, which is linked to faster cognitive decline. As with depression, social isolation might be a prodrome or a symptom of AD. Whatever the direction of causality, people who live alone, have never married, or are divorced or widowed have an increased risk of AD (Sundström et al. 2016). In a study of over 800,000 people, Sommerlad et al. (2017) found that being married is associated with reduced risk of about 40 percent compared with lifelong single people. Being widowed after extended co-habitation also took a toll, boosting the odds of AD by about 20 percent. They recommend that AD prevention in unmarried people should focus on education and physical health and should consider the possible effect of social engagement as a modifiable risk factor.

Diabetes

According to the American Diabetes Association, 27 percent of people aged 65 and older in the United States have diabetes and about half have pre-diabetes. Numerous studies have found that individuals with diabetes have a lower level of cognitive function and are at higher risk for AD than those without (Rawlings et al. 2014). Results presented at the 2015 Alzheimer's Association International Conference (AAIC) showed type-1 diabetics were 93 percent more likely to develop AD (73 percent after adjustment for heart health risk factors) than those without it. This suggests that diabetes prevention in the general population, as well as proper diabetes treatment in those who have been diagnosed, may have a role in preventing cognitive decline and AD (Luchsinger 2010). According to a 2011 study, nearly 175,000 cases of AD in the United States were attributable to diabetes, and a 25 percent reduction in diabetes prevalence could potentially have prevented 40,000 of these cases (Barnes and Yaffe 2011). The prevalence of diabetes in many countries, however, is increasing, threatening to reverse the apparent decline in AD rates in some HICs (Larson et al. 2013).

Hearing Loss

Hearing loss affects nearly a third of people over 55, but the idea that it may be a risk factor for AD is relatively recent (Lin and Albert 2014). The mechanism underlying cognitive decline associated with hearing loss is not yet clear, nor is it established whether corrections, such as hearing aids, can prevent or delay its onset, but there are several theories. One is that the extra effort required when people must struggle to hear may take away from the cognitive resources needed to successfully encode and preserve memories. The other is that hearing loss can lead to social disengagement, depression, and brain atrophy, all of which may accelerate cognitive decline.

Alcohol Abuse

Moderate to heavy alcohol consumption as risk factor for adverse brain outcomes and cognitive decline has long been assumed (Topiwala et al. 2017). A recent study confirmed that chronic heavy drinking is a robust risk factor for all types of dementia, especially early onset (Wise 2018). In this French study, researchers scrutinized the medical records of over a million adults diagnosed with dementia from 2008 to 2013 (Schwarzinger et al. 2018). They found that well over half the cases of early-onset dementia were either alcohol-related or accompanied by an additional diagnosis of alcohol abuse. Moreover, overall, alcohol disorders were associated with a three-fold heightened risk of all types of dementia. The link with alcohol was statistically unambiguous, leading the authors to suggest that screening, interventions for heavy drinking, and alcoholism treatment are needed to reduce cognitive decline. They concluded that the burden of dementia attributable to alcohol use disorders is much larger than previously thought.

Interventions Lacking Evidence of a Preventive Benefit

The NASEM study concluded that vitamin E, gingko biloba extract, and medications belonging to the class of anti-dementia drugs known as acetylcholinesterase inhibitors do not prevent or delay AD or improve cognitive function. Regarding the nutritional gingko biloba and vitamin E, the Committee notes that these supplements are widely marketed, with manufacturers claiming a variety of potential health benefits. While there is no evidence to suggest they are harmful, the cost of their purchase may not be justified if their intended use is to prevent cognitive decline or bolster cognitive performance. Trials of NSAIDs, estrogen hormone-replacement therapy, and statins also have been negative. Although hyperlipidemia is associated with cognitive decline (IOM 2015), there is no evidence that statins prevent or decrease cognitive impairment or AD.

As discussed in Chap. 3, a broad range of vitamin supplements and health food products are heavily touted and promoted as means of preventing cognitive impairment and, in some cases, reversing the effects of AD. To date, however, independent studies of the potential benefits of these products and medical foods for AD have not yielded positive results (Winblad et al. 2016). For instance, two multi-center RCTs showed no significant benefits of omega-3 fatty acid treatment on cognition, everyday activities, or global outcomes. Similarly, an independent study of Souvenaid concluded that it conferred no significant benefit on overall cognitive performance, and at best was associated with only very slight benefits on select areas of cognition, mainly memory. Nor did it offer any improvements in everyday functioning compared to a placebo (Scheltens et al. 2012).

Supplemental B vitamins (B_6, B_{12}, and folate) are of interest as possible interventions for preventing AD based on their ability to lower blood homocysteine levels, which, when elevated, are associated with increased risk of cardio- and cerebrovascular disease, as well as poor cognitive outcomes (IOM 2015). However, one review did not find any corroboration of benefits in cognitive function from B_{12} supplementation alone or in combination with other B vitamins (Ontario Health Technology Advisory Committee 2013). Similarly, the large Homocysteine and B Vitamins in Cognitive Impairment (VITACOG) study (Smith et al. 2010) examined vitamin B_6 and B_{12} and folic acid supplementation in 271 people with MCI. No significant benefit was found with respect to neuropsychological performance or the rate of brain atrophy. Further studies are needed to confirm if B vitamins and folic acid are beneficial in people with presymptomatic or pre-clinical AD and raised homocysteine concentrations (Livingston et al. 2017).

Vitamin E is the only other vitamin-based treatment with some clinical trial evidence of potential benefit. A significant and potentially important overall clinical benefit, equivalent to six months of natural decline, was shown for vitamin E compared with placebo for the primary outcome ADL. However, no benefit was reported for the group receiving both vitamin E and memantine, or for any of the secondary measures, including cognition (Dysken et al. 2014). Moreover, in one high-quality study, vitamin E did not reduce dementia or have any effect on a range of secondary outcomes (de Jager et al. 2012). Other RCTs of vitamin E have produced mixed results. Additionally, because the dose of vitamin E used in these studies is ten times higher than that usually sold as a food additive, potential safety issues need to be considered. For these reasons, the use of vitamin E as a clinical treatment for AD is not recommended at present (NASEM 2017).

Although there has been media interest in ketogenic treatments such as Axona, the only published clinical trial, a multi-center phase-2 RCT of 152 people with mild to moderate AD did not find any significant benefits on cognition or other outcomes after 90 days (Henderson et al. 2009). As introduced in Chap. 3, the theory that ketones could provide an alternative energy source for the brain is predicated on the unproven assumption that the brain's ability to use glucose is impaired in AD.

Importantly, the near lack of efficacy or safety evidence required for the marketing of all these supplements can not only create false expectations among consumers, but also could lead to health and safety issues. For example, beta-carotene, and vitamin E, as well as higher doses of vitamin A, seem to increase mortality (Bjelakovic et al. 2012). The authors conclude that anti-oxidant supplements need to be deemed medicinal products and should undergo sufficient evaluation before marketing. Another meta-analysis of RCTs reiterated that vitamin E supplementation is associated with increased mortality and an increased risk of hemorrhagic stroke (Schürks et al. 2010).

RESEARCH STRATEGIES FOR PUBLIC HEALTH AND ALZHEIMER'S

Public health strategies and plans to increase the diagnosis of AD are underway in many countries, including Denmark, France, Israel, the Netherlands, Norway, Switzerland, and the Britain. The British strategy consists of three parts (Department of Health 2013). First, was a public and practitioner information campaign, including television and newspaper advertisements to counter the argument that an AD diagnosis is of no benefit, rooted in the arguments that it is inevitable as one aged and that no treatment or support is available in any case. The second part was to provide practitioners with the tools to make a diagnosis and increase the number of diagnostic memory clinics (Burns and Robert 2009; Greaves and Jolly 2010). Finally, diagnosis rates were to be monitored and targeted at the primary care level with a goal to reach a two-thirds diagnosis rate. Since this strategy started, diagnosis rates in the UK have increased from less than 40 percent in 2009 to 67 percent in 2015, with a concomitant increase in the prescription of anti-dementia drugs

Similarly, both the NASEM and the Lancet Commission have called for major research initiatives on public health and AD. The NASEM argues that before funding research on preventing cognitive decline and dementia, the NIH and other interested organizations should improve the methodologies used by supporting studies that to all extent possible: identify individuals who are at higher risk of AD and tailor interventions accordingly; increase participation of underrepresented populations; begin interventions at younger ages and have longer follow-up periods; use consistent cognitive outcome measures to enable pooling; include biomarkers as intermediate outcomes; and conduct large trials designed to test the effectiveness of an intervention in broad, routine clinical practices or community settings.

A high priority for AD research is to strengthen the evidence base for those interventions that currently have insufficient evidence to determine their effectiveness: new anti-dementia treatments that can delay onset or slow disease progression, diabetes and depression treatment, dietary interventions, lipid-lowering treatment/statins, sleep quality interventions, social engagement interventions, and vitamin B_{12} plus folic acid supplementation. Although inconclusive, clinical trials and other studies have yielded encouraging data for some interventions, and the public should have access to this information to inform choices on how to invest time and resources to maintain brain health with aging.

One pertinent issue when pursuing a public health approach to AD is the extent to which it is ethical to tap into the fear of dementia discussed in Chap. 3. Should the public's fear of developing AD be used in public health campaigns to encourage health initiatives that are found to be effective in preventing it? In other words, should we use a fear-based approach, as is done with tobacco use by utilizing graphic ads that illustrate the dangers of smoking, or will this be interpreted as further stigmatizing people with AD? Chapter 6 turns attention to the many issues surrounding AD at the end of life.

REFERENCES

AARP (2017) Global Council on Brain Health. http://www.aarp.org/health/brain-health/global-council-on-brain-health.

Alzheimer Europe (2016) National Dementia Strategies. http://alzheimer-europe.org/Policy-in-Practice2/National-Dementia-Strategies/.

Alzheimer's Impact Movement (2018) "BOLD Infrastructure for Alzheimer's Act." https://alzimpact.org/priorities/bold_alzheimers_act?WT.mc_id=enews2018_04_04&utm_source=enews-aff-38&utm_medium=email&utm_campaign=enews-2018-04-04.

Barnes, D.E. and K. Yaffe (2011) "The projected effect of risk factor reduction on Alzheimer's disease prevalence." *The Lancet Neurology* 10 (9): 819–28.

Baumgart, M., H.M. Snyder, M.C. Carrillo, S. Fazio et al. (2015) "Summary of the evidence on modifiable risk factors for cognitive decline and dementia: A population-based perspective." *Alzheimer's & Dementia: The Journal of the Alzheimer's Association* 11 (6): 718–26.

Bjelakovic, G., D. Nikolova, L.L. Gluud, R.G. Simonetti and C. Gluud (2012) "Antioxidant supplements for prevention of mortality in healthy participants and patients with various diseases." *Cochrane Database Systems Review* 14 (3): CD007176. https://doi.org/10.1002/14651858.CD007176.pub2.

Borenstein, A. and J. Mortimer (2016) *Alzheimer's Disease: Life Course Perspectives on Risk Reduction.* Cambridge, MA: Academic Press.

Burns, A. and P. Robert (2009) "The national dementia strategy in England." *British Medical Journal* 338: b931.

Chirles, T.J., K. Reiter, L.R. Weiss, A.J. Alfini et al. (2017) "Exercise training and functional connectivity changes in mild cognitive impairment and healthy elders." *Journal of Alzheimer's Disease* 57 (3): 845–56. https://doi.org/10.3233/JAD-161151.

Cholerton, B., E.B. Larson, L.D. Baker et al. (2013) "Neuropathologic correlates of cognition in a population-based sample." *Journal of Alzheimer's Disease* 36: 699–709

Dalton, A.M., N. Wareham, S. Griffin and A.P. Jones (2016) "Neighbourhood greenspace is associated with a slower decline in physical activity in older adults: A prospective cohort study." *SSM—Population Health* 2: 683–91.

de Jager, C.A., A. Oulhaj, R. Jacoby, H. Refsum and A.D. Smith (2012) "Cognitive and clinical outcomes of homocysteine-lowering B-vitamin treatment in mild cognitive impairment: A randomized controlled trial." *International Journal of Geriatric Psychiatry* 27: 592–600.

Department of Health (2013) *Dementia: A State of the Nation Report on Dementia Care and Support in England.* London: Department of Health.

Dysken, M.W., M. Sano, S. Asthana, J.E. Vertrees et al. (2014) "Effect of vitamin E and memantine on functional decline in Alzheimer disease: The TEAM-AD VA cooperative randomized trial." *Journal of the American Medical Association* 311: 33–44.

Forlini, C. and W. Hall (2017) "A prospectus for ethical analysis of ageing individuals' responsibility to prevent cognitive decline." *Bioethics.* https://doi.org/10.1111/bioe.12387.

Frankish, H. and R. Horton (2017) "Prevention and management of dementia: A priority for public health." *The Lancet.* https://doi.org/10.1016/S0140-6736(17)31756-7.

Greaves, I. and D. Jolly (2010) "National dementia strategy: Well intentioned, but how well founded and how well directed?" *British Journal of General Practice* 60 (572): 193–98.

G-Science Academiers (2016) "G-Science Academies statement 2016: Understanding, protecting, and developing global brain resources." http://fpcj.

jp/wp/wp-content/uploads/2016/05/3Three-Joint-Statements-of-G-Science-Academies-2016.pdf.

Henderson, S.T., J.L. Vogel, L.J. Barr, F. Garvin et al. (2009) "Study of the ketogenic agent AC-1202 in mild to moderate Alzheimer's disease: A randomized, double-blind, placebo-controlled, multicenter trial." *Nutrition and Metabolism* 6: 31.

Hörder, H., L. Johansson, X-X. Guo and G. Grimby (2018) "Midlife cardiovascular fitness and dementia A 44-year longitudinal population study in women." *Neurology.* https://doi.org/10.1212/WNL.0000000000005290.

Innes, A. and B. Director (2013) "Working towards dementia friendly societies." *Perspectives in Public Health* 133 (3): 141.

IOM (Institute of Medicine) (2015) *Cognitive Aging: Progress in Understanding and Opportunities for Action.* Washington, DC: The National Academies Press.

Kane, R.L., M. Butler, H.A. Fink, M. Brasure et al. (2017) "Interventions to prevent age-related cognitive decline, mild cognitive impairment, and clinical Alzheimer's-type dementia." Comparative Effectiveness Review 188. Rockville, MD: Agency for Healthcare Research and Quality.

Larson, E.B. and K.M. Langa (2017) "What's the "take home" from research on dementia trends." *PLoS Medicine* 14 (3): e1002236.

Larson, E.B., K. Yaffe, and K.M. Langa (2013) "New insights into the dementia epidemic." *New England Journal of Medicine* 369 (24): 2275–77.

Lin, F.R. and M. Albert (2014) "Hearing loss and dementia—Who is listening?" *Aging Mental Health* 18: 671–73.

Livingston, G., A. Sommerlad, V. Orgeta, S.G. Costafreda et al. (2017) "Dementia prevention, intervention, and care." *The Lancet.* https://doi.org/10.1016/S0140-6736(17)31363-6.

Luchsinger, J.A. (2010) "Diabetes, related conditions, and dementia." *Journal of the Neurological Sciences* 299 (1–2): 35–38.

Mayeda, E.R., M.M. Glymour, C.P. Quesenberry and R.A. Whitmer (2014) "Inequalities in dementia incidence between six racial and ethnic groups over 14 years." *Alzheimer's & Dementia: The Journal of the Alzheimer's Association* 12 (3): 216–24.

Meng, X. and C. D'Arcy (2012) "Education and dementia in the context of the cognitive reserve hypothesis: A systematic review with meta-analyses and qualitative analyses." *PLoS ONE* 7: e38268.

Moll van Charante, E.P., E. Richard, L.S. Eurelings, J.W. van Dalen et al. (2016) "Effectiveness of a 6-year multidomain vascular care intervention to prevent dementia (preDIVA): A cluster-randomised controlled trial." *Lancet* 388: 797–805.

National Academies of Sciences, Engineering, and Medicine (NASEM) (2017) *Preventing Cognitive Decline and Dementia: A Way Forward.* Washington, DC: The National Academies Press.

Norton, S., F.E. Matthews, D.E. Barnes, K. Yaffe and C. Brayne (2014) "Potential for primary prevention of Alzheimer's disease: An analysis of population-based data." *Lancet Neurology* 13: 788–94.

Ontario Health Technology Assessment Committee (2013) "Vitamin B12 and cognitive function: An evidencebased analysis." *Ontario Health Technology Assessment Service* 13 (23): 1–45.

Panza, G.A., B.A. Taylor, H.V. MacDonald, B.T. Johnson et al. (2018) "Can exercise improve cognitive symptoms of Alzheimer's disease? A meta-analysis." *Journal of the American Geriatrics Society.* https://doi.org/10.1111/jgs.15241.

Prince, M.J. (2017) "Progress on dementia—Leaving no one behind." *The Lancet.* https://doi.org/10.1016/S0140-6736(17)31757-9.

Prince, M.J., G.C. Ali, M. Guerchet, A.M. Prina et al. (2016) "Recent global trends in the prevalence and incidence of dementia, and survival with dementia." *Alzheimer's Research and Therapy* 8: 23. https://doi.org/10.1186/s13195-016-0188-8.

Qizilbash, N., J. Gregson, M.E. Johnson, N. Pearce et al. (2015) "BMI and risk of dementia in two million people over two decades: A retrospective cohort study." *The Lancet: Diabetes and Endocrinology* 3 (6): 431–36.

Rahimi, J. and G.G. Kovacs (2014) "Prevalence of mixed pathologies in the aging brain." *Alzheimer's Research and Therapy* 6 (9): 82–89.

Rawlings, A.M., A.R. Sharrett, A.L.C. Schneider, J. Coresh, M. Albert et al. (2014) "Diabetes in midlife and cognitive change over 20 years: The Atherosclerosis Risk in Communities Neurocognitive Study." *Annals of Internal Medicine* 161 (11): 785–93.

Ritchie, K., C.W. Ritchie, K. Yaffe, I. Skoog, and N. Scarmeas (2015) "Is late-onset Alzheimer's disease really a disease of midlife?" *Alzheimer's and Dementia: Translational Research and Clinical Interventions* 1 (2): 122–30.

Satizabal, C.L., A.S. Beiser, V. Chouraki, G. Chêne et al. (2016) "Incidence of dementia over three decades in the Framingham Heart Study." *New England Journal of Medicine* 374: 523–32.

Scheltens, P., T.W. Twisk, R. Blesa, E. Scarpini et al. (2012) "Efficacy of Souvenaid in mild Alzheimer's disease: Results from a randomized, controlled trial." *Journal of Alzheimer's Disease* 31: 225–36.

Schürks, M., R.J. Glynn, P.M. Rist, C. Tzourio and T. Kurth (2010) "Effects of vitamin E on stroke subtypes: Meta-analysis of randomised controlled trials." *British Medical Journal* 341: c5702.

Schwarzinger, M., B.G. Pollock, O.S.M. Hasan, C. Dufouil and J. Rehm (2018) "Contribution of alcohol use disorders to the burden of dementia in France 2008–13: A nationwide retrospective cohort study." *The Lancet Public Health.* https://doi.org/10.1016/S2468-2667(18)30022-7.

Smith, A.D., S.M. Smith, C.A. de Jager et al. (2010) "Homocysteine-lowering by B vitamins slows the rate of accelerated brain atrophy in mild cognitive impairment: A randomized controlled trial." *PLoS ONE* 5: e12244.

Sofi, F., D. Valecchi, D. Bacci et al. (2011) "Physical activity and risk of cognitive decline: A meta-analysis of prospective studies." *Journal of Internal Medicine* 269: 107–17.

Sommerlad, A., J. Ruegger, A. Singh-Manoux, G. Lewis and G. Livingston (2017) "Marriage and risk of dementia: Systematic review and meta-analysis of observational studies." *Journal of Neurology, Neurosurgery and Psychiatry.* https://doi.org/10.1136/jnnp-2017-316274.

Sundström, A., O. Westerlund and E. Kotyrlo (2016) "Marital status and risk of dementia: A nationwide population-based prospective study from Sweden." *BMJ Open* 6: e008565.

ten Brinke, L.F., N. Bolandzadeh, L.S. Nagamatsu, C.L. Hsu et al. (2017) "Aerobic exercise increases hippocampal volume in older women with probable mild cognitive impairment: A 6-month randomised controlled trial." *British Journal of Sports Medicine* 49 (4): https://doi.org/10.1136/bjsports-2013-093184.

Topiwala, A, C.L. Allan, V. Valkanova et al. (2017) "Moderate alcohol consumption as risk factor for adverse brain outcomes and cognitive decline: Longitudinal cohort study." *British Medical Journal* 357: j2353.

Winblad, B., P. Amouyel, S. Andrieu, C. Ballard et al. (2016) "Defeating Alzheimer's disease and other dementias: A priority for European science and society." *Lancet Neurology* 15: 455–532.

Wise, J. (2018) "Large study is 'robust' evidence of link between chronic heavy drinking and dementia." *British Medical Journal* 360: k814.

WHO (2017) Draft global action plan on the public health response to dementia. Report by the Director-General. April 3. http://apps.who.int/gb/ebwha/pdf_files/WHA70/A70_28-en.pdf?ua=1 (Accessed June 26, 2017).

Yaffe, K., C. Falvey, T.B. Harris, A. Newman et al. (2013) "Effect of socioeconomic disparities on incidence of dementia among biracial older adults: Prospective study." *British Medical Journal* 347: f7051.

Young, J., M. Angevaren, J. Rusted and N. Tabet (2015) "Aerobic exercise to improve cognitive function in older people without known cognitive impairment." *Cochrane Database System Review* 4: CD005381.

CHAPTER 6

End-of-Life Decision Making for Alzheimer's Disease Across Cultures

Abstract This chapter discusses a range of policy and ethical issues dealing with end-of-life decision making for Alzheimer's patients. It analyzes issues including: palliative care; advance directives; withholding or withdrawing artificial hydration and feeding, antibiotics, and other care; and physician-assisted suicide. Caring for someone with AD at the end of life raises unique challenges because, in contrast to cancer and other advanced chronic diseases, a person with AD at some stage will lose cognitive abilities, function, and capacity. Therefore, they will be unable to make decisions about their care and treatment or express their needs and wishes for a protracted period as death approaches. This chapter also reviews the wide variation of end-of-life policies across cultures and within the United States.

Keywords End-of-life decision making • Palliative care • Euthanasia • Ethical issues

In recent years, end-of-life decision making has engendered a vigorous dialogue because it raises broad and difficult ethical issues that impact health professionals, patients, and their families. This concern is exacerbated by the high costs related to end-of-life care especially in the United States. Historically, death and the dying process were largely a matter of

© The Author(s) 2019   121
R. H. Blank, *Social & Public Policy of Alzheimer's Disease in the United States*, https://doi.org/10.1007/978-981-13-0656-3_6

private decisions made within specific religious and cultural frameworks; however, because of demographic trends and an expanding array of life-saving technologies leading to progressively scarce health care resources, how we make these decisions has become a matter of public policy and ethical debate. As a growing proportion of societal resources are becoming concentrated at the end of life, the issues will intensify.

There are numerous overlapping issues that together define the context of policy making at the end of life. Basic questions relate to what institutional services exist for care of the critically or terminally ill; how, where, and by whom these patients are treated; and who makes the final decisions as to level of care given? Do individuals generally die in intensive care units, hospital wards, nursing homes, hospices or at home? In addition, what, if any, boundaries or cut-off points exist for aggressive treatment of a specific patient and under what circumstances are cardiopulmonary resuscitation (CPR) and artificial hydration and nutrition used? Moreover, how is such care funded and who ultimately makes the life-ending decision in cases where the patient is unable to so: doctors, the family, ethics committees, the government, or some combination?

Accompanying the medical dimensions of policy making at the end of life are the social and legal aspects. In many Western countries, considerable emphasis recently has been directed toward empowerment of the patient or patient autonomy. A wide variety of legal mechanisms have been created toward this end in some countries, but by no means most. The stated goal of advance directives, whether living wills or powers of attorney, is to return to the individual the ability to control the dying process, primarily by refusing life-extending interventions, but this is far from universally accepted. There are conflicting views on the effectiveness of advance directives especially for AD patients, and cultural factors have produced divergent views on their use even where legal.

Related to advance directives are various policy initiatives over the concept of euthanasia, itself loaded with complex and varied meanings both within and across cultures and countries. Some commentators distinguish between passive and active, voluntary and involuntary, and other categories of euthanasia, thus allowing for support of some, but not other, types. Others argue that such distinctions are artificial and that all forms of euthanasia are morally wrong and should be outlawed. Still others argue that the distinctions are meaningless and that individuals should not be precluded by law or moral codes from making their own choice as to how and when to die. Although the most vehement opposition to euthanasia tends to center on those cases where active assistance of a third party is required, the debate over physician-assisted suicide (PAS) frequently is deliberately linked with cases involving the withholding or withdrawing of treatment, thus again clouding the lines between passive and active types. The question remains as to how political systems should define and deal with withholding or withdrawing specific types of intervention or with more direct forms of termination of life in cases of advanced AD.

Most research on end-of-life care for AD has focused on those in the advanced stage rather than those with less severe dementia who are dying from other conditions (Livingston et al. 2017). Caring for someone with AD at the end of life raises unique challenges. In contrast to cancer and other advanced chronic diseases, a person with AD at some stage will lose cognitive abilities, function, and capacity. Therefore, they will be unable to make decisions about their care and treatment or express their needs and wishes for a protracted period as death approaches. Moreover, because substantial prognostic uncertainty exists, the course of AD is unpredictable. However, most end-stage AD patients experience an array of symptoms including pressure sores, agitation, swallowing difficulties, and depression, some of which might be poorly detected and thus undertreated. They are often immobile, bed bound, at risk of aspiration, and have an impaired immunological function that heightens their risk of pneumonia, urinary tract, and other infections (van der Steen et al. 2009). Lack of proper assessment and management of pain can lead to reduced quality of life, depression, worsening agitation, and other neuropsychiatric symptoms (Lichtner et al. 2014). Additionally, distress and discomfort can be exacerbated by room temperature, poor positioning, boredom, and lack of social contact.

PALLIATIVE CARE FOR AD PATIENTS AT END OF LIFE

The Lancet Commission argues that we should focus on maximizing comfort and quality of life, rather than developing strict criteria as to when the AD patient can access hospice care (Livingston et al. 2017). Control of pain and other symptoms of psychological, social, and spiritual problems is paramount. The goal of palliative care is achievement of the best quality of life for patients and their families. The European Association of Palliative Care acknowledges the vital role of caregivers and family members who might experience distress and anticipatory grief since they must make difficult, emotionally demanding choices as death approaches.

Until recently, often those dying from end-stage AD have not been viewed as having a terminal condition and were less likely than others to be managed palliatively (ADI 2016). However, US nursing homes are moving toward providing a more palliative approach to end-of-life care for residents with AD. Liu et al. (2015) compared the use of hospice care in the last 100 days of life for over a million nursing home deaths between 2003 and 2007. Over that period, hospice use for people dying with AD increased from 25.1 to 36.5 percent as compared to 26.5 to 34.4 percent for those without AD, while the rate of in-hospital deaths remained virtually unchanged. By 2007, people dying with AD were more likely than others to use hospice care services and significantly less likely to die in a hospital. In a study of those admitted to hospice care, the quality of care for those with a diagnosis of AD did not differ from those without except with respect to an excess use of tube-feeding (Albrecht et al. 2013). Likewise, a Dutch End of Life in Dementia study confirmed that appropriate palliative care measures were prevalent in nursing homes for AD patients during the last week of life. Pain and shortness of breath were mostly treated with opioids and agitation mainly with anxiolytics while bronchodilators and diuretics were used for symptomatic relief. On the day of death, 77 percent were receiving opioids and 21 percent palliative sedation (Hendriks et al. 2014).

According to ADI (2016), good quality end-of-life care concerns attention to symptom burden that for people with AD is a common problem. Achieving comfort may require intensive medical management and pharmacological as well as non-pharmacological intervention, in conjunction with avoidance of futile and burdensome interventions. In the Dutch study, the most common symptoms in the last week of life for nursing home residents were pain (52 percent), followed by agitation (35 percent), and shortness of breath (35 percent) (Hendriks et al. 2014). Pain and agitation, especially, were strongly associated with low quality of life. Death from respiratory infection was associated with the largest symptom burden. Because of communication difficulties in advanced AD and a lack of good assessment skills by some health professionals, some of the symptoms including pain are underdetected in patients with AD (Sampson 2010). Although underdetection can lead to undertreatment of symptoms, alternatively, overtreatment with burdensome and futile interventions, such as tube-feeding and antibiotics, should be avoided (van der Steen 2010).

In a German poll of caregivers, 43 percent of those with AD (compared with 36 percent of others) died at home, which was the preferred outcome for 95 percent of patients and 78 percent of the caregivers (Pinzon et al. 2013). This confirms that, unless they have pain or distress that cannot be treated, most people with AD prefer to die in their usual place of residence. Improved continuity of care could also decrease costs by reducing emergency room visits and hospital admissions, which seldom prolong life and can be distressing (Livingston et al. 2017). Pinzon and associates found that, according to caregivers, most AD patients suffered in the days before death from symptoms that could have been alleviated. For people with AD, end-of-life care at home and in care homes was rated better than hospital care, with caregivers especially critical of the quality of care received on hospital wards, often citing a limited availability of staff and emotional support (Pinzon et al. 2013; Davies et al. 2014). Key elements include frequency of contact, provision of information, and support and reassurance for the caregivers. Moreover, support for caregivers should be culturally sensitive and account for ethnic differences in caregiving experiences, attitudes to end-of-life care, and bereavement reactions (Owen et al. 2001).

Alzheimer Europe (2008) guidelines highlight the common complaint of caregivers that they are excluded or that the AD patient is not being cared for properly when care is taken over by professionals as additional medical and nursing support is required. Caregivers often feel that they are best placed to understand the needs and wishes of the patient and want to share this with the health care professionals. Alzheimer Europe recommends that a good relationship and an atmosphere of trust are established when caregivers' concerns and criticisms are dealt with in a positive manner and they are given an opportunity to participate in the care process. When care is provided at a hospital or nursing home, caregivers may want to be continuously present, and this need should be met with the possibility to sleep at the facility. For those dying at home, flexible respite care allows caregivers to get breaks with the reassurance that they will be with the patient at the time of death.

In Britain, the Appreciative Inquiry on service and hospital care costs for AD patients living in care homes was assessed for three care homes before and after implementation of the six-month intervention. It aimed to change how care home staff, primary care practitioners, and nurses worked together to address difficulties and uncertainties of providing end-of-life care to AD patients (Amador et al. 2014). Following the intervention, total service costs fell by 43 percent and hospital care costs by 88 percent. Similarly, in New York, pharmacy costs were compared before and after a palliative care consultation for 60 hospital in-patients with advanced AD (Araw et al. 2015). Although there was a decrease in overall average daily pharmacy cost from US$31.16 to $20.83, it was matched by an increase in the proportion of participants taking analgesics and a proportionate rise in daily analgesic cost.

Legal, Ethical, and Policy Issues at the End of Life

The realities of AD progression, fueled by the fear of AD because of its impact on personal autonomy, have led to considerable apprehension as to how best a person can maintain control over their dying process. This, in turn, has led to a wide array of legal and policy issues including:

- Advance directives and other proxy documents
- Withholding respirators and other mechanical support
- Withholding feeding or hydration tubes
- Withholding antibiotics
- Withdrawing any of the above
- Palliative care—hospice
- Suicide and assisted suicide

Table 6.1 illustrates the possible categories of end-of-life decisions. Passive measures include decisions to withhold or withdraw treatments that might extend a patient's life, while active measures involve direct inducement of death by either providing the means of ending life or assisting in it. Importantly, these decisions can be voluntary on the part of a competent patient, speculative, or involuntary against the explicit wishes of the patient. Although passive involuntary could include policies of rationing that deny life-saving resources, involuntary active decisions are at present inconceivable in democracies. Because of the problems discussed above, most such decisions for AD patients fall in the speculative category and will always be disputable (Smith 2013).

Advance Directives and Treatment Options

Although there has been a trend toward increased acceptance of advance directives for AD patients, they are especially difficult because they involve the authority of the former competent self to govern the life of the later,

Table 6.1   Categories of end-of-life decisions

	Passive *Omission of measures to* *prolong life*	*Active* *Direct inducement of death*
Voluntary With patient's express and informed consent.	*Passive Voluntary:* Conscious *and* rational patient refuses life- prolonging treatment and request is granted.	*Active Voluntary:* Conscious *and* rational patient requests and is given help to cause death, usually a lethal injection.
Speculative Without express and informed consent (i.e., comatose patient, infant, dementia patient).	*Passive Speculative:* Cessation of life-prolonging treatment for patient unable to give informed consent.	*Active Speculative:* Lethal injection administered to patient unable to give informed consent.
Involuntary Against the express directions of the patient.	*Passive Involuntary:* Cessation of life-prolonging treatment to conscious and rational person against her will.	*Active Involuntary:* Lethal injections administered to conscious and rational patient against his will.

Source: Blank (1995: 163)

non-competent self. Critics of advance directives highlight the difficulties in projecting decisions to future states or personal identities of selves that may be drastically different because of physical or mental changes brought on by AD. Furthermore, if the directive includes choosing a proxy, this can result in proxies projecting their own values onto various possible future circumstances when they make decisions for the person. This is problematic because caregivers tend to report lower scores on quality of life than the patients themselves (Hertogh 2005). Moreover, Tomlinson and Stott (2014) found that health professionals hold more restrictive views toward assisted dying than patients, the public, and carers.

Advance directives must be made soon after diagnosis when the person with AD still has the level of judgment and decision-making capacity necessary to sign official documents or make medical decisions. Whatever instrument is used, it is important that one understands the range of treatment options available when making decisions to use, withdraw, limit, or refuse treatment, especially in the late stage of the disease when they are no longer competent (Alzheimer's Association 2016).

The use of artificial nutrition and hydration (including intravenous fluids and parenteral feeding) in advanced AD is controversial because there is little evidence that they reduce the risk of aspiration pneumonia, prolong life, or even improve nutritional status or quality of life (Livingston et al. 2017). Moreover, they can result in infections and the need for physical restraints. In fact, a lack of hydration is a normal part of the dying process and can allow a more comfortable death over a period of days. Furthermore, difficulty swallowing and decreased appetite, sometimes secondary to lower caloric requirements, are common features of end-stage AD. Families might be concerned that their relative is hungry or thirsty, and helping with eating is often a way to enact their care for their relative. Practices about using percutaneous endoscopic gastrostomy and nasogastric tubes varies among countries (Wada et al. 2014) and even across US states due to legal differences (Ahronheim et al. 2001).

Antibiotics may be prescribed to treat infections, such as pneumonia and urinary tract, that are common with late-stage AD, but they are unlikely to improve the patient's condition. Prior to the availability of antibiotics, pneumonia was often seen as a welcome form of death. Moreover, although a respirator can help keep alive a person who cannot breathe on their own, it can cause the body to undergo unneeded stress and great discomfort. Thus, many experts discourage CPR for terminally ill patients as it can be painful and traumatic, might leave the person worse off, and is unlikely to prolong life. A do-not-resuscitate (DNR) order states that no attempts will be made to revive the person and is commonplace for most advanced AD patients, although again it varies by culture.

The Alzheimer's Association emphasizes that refusal or withdrawal of treatment, including tube-feeding, antibiotics, CPR, or other treatments, does not constitute assisted suicide (Alzheimer's Association 2016). Limiting treatment lets the disease take its natural course and supports the person's comfort and dignity. If aggressive medical treatment is refused or withdrawn, a care team should still provide comprehensive physical and emotional care. Instead of seeking a cure or trying to prolong life, palliative care focuses on dignity and quality of remaining life by keeping the person comfortable and pain-free until life ends. It usually excludes medical treatments, tests, and procedures that might cause discomfort.

Suicide and Euthanasia of AD Patients across Cultures

In the absence of effective treatments for AD, there is evidence that persons with MCI and early AD are at heightened risk for suicide or for requesting PAS (Draper et al. 2010). Barak and Aizenberg (2002) note that suicide attempts are not rare in elderly patients with AD, especially among those with higher levels of daily functioning. The ensuing clinical, ethical, and legal dilemmas associated with PAS in the context of AD are a subject of intense debate (Humphry 2014). Clearly, diagnosis has different meanings for different people, who can experience a range of possible reactions. Rabins (2007) notes that although about 60 percent of those with AD are unaware that they have a problem and remain unconvinced of any problem when they are diagnosed, for some, the emotional adjustment is so overwhelming that suicide ensues within months of diagnosis.

PAS, or active euthanasia, is the active and deliberate termination of a patient's life at the explicit request of a patient. Although such practices are highly controversial and illegal in most countries, the laws are more liberal in Belgium, Switzerland, the Netherlands, and an increasing number of US states, such as Oregon, Washington, California, and Colorado. The first state to allow PAS, Oregon, operates under very strict controls and has an annual number of assisted deaths reported less than 50. In 2016, Canada federal legislation permitted PAS for patients with a "serious and incurable illness, disease, or disability" that causes intolerable suffering where death was "reasonably foreseeable." In the Netherlands, under the Euthanasia Act of 2002, PAS is legally justified for terminal patents only if the physician is satisfied that the patient's request is voluntary, well considered, sustained, and well informed, and that the person is fully competent at the time of the request and views his or her situation as one of unbearable or hopeless suffering. Even with these restrictions, however, PAS remains controversial and is still not an established practice without legal implications (Miller et al. 2018).

Most experts believe that patients with AD cannot satisfy the letter of these criteria and, thus, are ineligible for PAS as the laws are currently written (Hertogh 2005). When patients are competent to make the decision to end their lives, they often have significantly longer than six months left to live, but by the time they have less than six months to live, they are no longer legally competent (Guidry 2014). Although in theory the Dutch law supports the possibility of having the request substituted by an advance directive, in practice, this option is difficult to realize, because while an advance directive presupposes a very careful and detailed statement of the wishes, most are unspecific. Also, most doctors find it unacceptable to perform PAS on a person who cannot at that moment express his or her will or even understand what the physician is about to do (de Beaufort and van de Vathorst 2016). Miller and Appelbaum (2018), however, note that physicians in the Netherlands and Belgium have helped a small but grow-ing number of patients with mental illness but no terminal condition to end their lives and that in some US states attempts to extend PAS to psy-chiatric patients appear inevitable.

Although PAS remains illegal in most jurisdictions, there has been a trend toward acceptance or at least tolerance of other forms of euthanasia, particularly the withholding of medical technologies. Again, culture and the sophistication and availability of medical technologies in a country appear to be major influences (Blank and Merrick 2007). Given the fear of AD, it is not surprising that in countries where PAS is legal, a growing number of people are initiating advance directives in which they express the desire to terminate their lives at some stage of the disease. In countries where PAS is illegal, clinical experience and anecdotal reports suggest that people are making covert arrangements for some form of assisted suicide in the event of being diagnosed with AD (Draper et al. 2010). In the Netherlands in 2014, 81 people diagnosed with AD were granted eutha-nasia and their doctors either administered lethal drugs on their request or helped them by providing the drugs (de Beaufort and van de Vathorst 2016). Almost all these cases involved persons who were in the early stages of the disease and were considered competent and still able to make an autonomous choice. Having to decide, while still competent, however, may mean that people die earlier than even they might have preferred, because waiting entails the risk that they will be judged to be incompetent, and then the opportunity will be lost.

Prosporo rejects the practice of letting an arbitrary infection determine the death of a patient that puts the patient and family through unnecessary suffering (Prosporo 2015). Because infections have varying degrees of severity in how quickly they may be fatal or the pain they incur, he argues that PAS with advance directive is the most caring means of respecting the interests of patients with end-stage AD. Since AD destroys the neurobio-logical basis for the access consciousness necessary for moral capacity, the formerly expressed interest should be respected. AD patients are vulnera-ble to be in Catch 22 situation because of the difficulty, if not inability, to express their own interests.

An oft-cited threat to the voluntariness of a choice of euthanasia for AD patients is the possibility of pressure from family or from society leading to feelings of a duty to die or to guilt about being a burden (Smith 2013). If AD patients are covertly or overtly given the impression that they are a burden to their families and/or society in general, then their requests to die might not be fully voluntary. In general, those who have severe AD are unable to initiate or carry out the act of killing themselves. Thus, some observers consider it rational, or at least understandable, for people with less advanced AD to take their own lives even if their quality of life is still good, with the knowledge that in due course (although maybe not for years) they will lack the capacity to effect their own suicide (Smith 2013). It is not necessarily the end state of total dependence that is feared, then, but the loss of mental faculties that begin in the earlier stages of the disease that will ultimately take away their legal choices (McCrae 2014). For instance, the first person to die using Kevorkian's "suicide machine" was a 54-year-old woman with early-onset AD, who persuaded him that her decision was rational and the result of long and careful reflection. Similarly, in 2011, a 64-year-old woman, who had declared for several years that she wanted to be euthanized, was the first documented case of a person with advanced AD to undergo PAS in the Netherlands (Kouwenhoven et al. 2015).

The first reported case of a British citizen using PAS took place at Dignitas Assisted Suicide Centre in Switzerland in 2013. The 83-year-old man was in the early stages of AD and wanted to avoid the debilitating process and make certain that his family did not see him suffer. In a survey of British adults at the time, 55 percent agreed to a PAS for mild and moderate cases and 60 percent for severe cases of AD. The assisted dying campaign has focused not on pain alleviation but on perceived loss of dignity. The Kantian view is that dignity derives from autonomy, but this deprives people with advanced AD of a defining quality of human life. An unintended consequence of this rationale for euthanasia is to imply that AD at the end stage is undignified. McCrae and Bloomfield (2013) warn that this perception could extend to AD overall, devaluing the status of people with it and perpetuating the poor standards of care often found in institutional settings.

Johnstone decries the "Alzheimerization" of the euthanasia debate, arguing that the way AD is portrayed by advocacy groups and the media as the disease that is poised to have a near-catastrophic impact on the world's health care system is having undue influence on the euthanasia debate (Johnstone 2013). This representation of the disease makes AD a "soft target" in the euthanasia debate because it plays to people's fears of developing the disease and what it symbolizes. It positions AD as something that requires a remedy, that remedy increasingly being pre-emptive and beneficent euthanasia. Johnstone acknowledges that euthanasia is a polarizing and emotive issue; however, she warns that the public can be unduly swayed by the way the media and pro-euthanasia groups frame the issue as simply a matter of choice often through highly personalized, individual experiences.

IMPORTANCE OF CULTURE AND RELIGION

End-of-life decision making remains a highly emotional and divisive policy area with strong cultural and religious undercurrents. Cox et al. (2006) conclude that there are significant cultural differences regarding advance care planning and end-of-life decision making that present major challenges for health care providers. For instance, advance directives, which are generally accepted in the West, hold little or no relevance in other cultures. Similarly, for the most part, only in the United States do we consider artificially feeding patients with AD or feel that we are starving a patient to death by withholding it. "Curiously, many cultures see stopping eating as a sign of dying and not its cause. They never even consider the use of a feeding tube" (Dunn 2009).

Likewise, Searight and Gafford (2005) argue that the US model of health care that values autonomy in medical decision making is not easily applied to some racial and ethnic groups. There remain major differences across cultures regarding communication of bad news, the locus of decisions, and attitudes toward advance directives. Thus, in contrast to the emphasis on truth telling in the United States, health care professionals in other countries frequently conceal critical diagnoses from patients out of deference to respect or potential harm to the patient. It is common practice in Asian cultures for health care providers not to disclose the truth of an illness (Searight and Gafford 2005). The responsibility of telling is left to the family, but often mutual silence prevails between patients and families when discussing medical issues and a lack of communication persists.

Although the Asian cultures might be most divergent from Western values, there is considerable variation within the West as well. In a major study of decisions by patients, families, and health care providers about medical care at the end of life in 37 European ICUs, culture was found to have a major impact on end-of-life policy across Europe. Decisions regarding CPR, withholding or withdrawing treatment, and active shortening of the dying process all reflected statistically significant differences among regions that could be attributed largely to cultural factors (Cohen et al. 2005). Another study, drawn from the same data set, found that withholding occurred more often than withdrawing if the physician was Jewish, Greek Orthodox, or Muslim, while withdrawing occurred more often for physicians who were Catholic, Protestant, or had no religious affiliation (Sprung et al. 2007).

Moreover, given increased cultural diversity within Western nations, there can be strong cultural and value divisions within each country that are important in defining end-of-life policies for AD patients. In addition, social structures, particularly the importance of the family and the role of women, can be central to care of end-stage AD patients and in setting the boundaries of such care. Even within the United States there are significant differences by race. One study concluded that a large majority of seriously ill older Latinos favored family-centered decisions and limited patient autonomy (Kelley et al. 2010), while another found that values of denial, secrecy about prognosis, and a collective, family-centered system lowered hospice use by Latinos (Heyman and Gutheil 2010). Furthermore, African-American patients generally are more desirous of life-sustaining treatment than comparable whites; they are more likely to demand all available measures to save a life irrespective of illness severity; and largely reject any form of assisted death (Shrank et al. 2005). These intra-societal divisions are bound to complicate even further end-of-life policy making for people with AD.

References

Ahronheim, J.C., M. Mulvihill, C. Sieger, P. Park and B.E. Fries (2001) "State practice variations in the use of tube feeding for nursing home residents with severe cognitive impairment." *Journal of the American Geriatric Society* 49: 148–52.

Albrecht, J.S., A.L. Gruber-Baldini, E.K. Fromme, J.C. McGregor, D.S. Lee and J.P. Furuno (2013) "Quality of hospice care for individuals with dementia." *Journal of the American Geriatric Society* 61 (7): 1060–5.

Alzheimer's Association (2016) End-of-life decisions: Honoring the wishes of a person with Alzheimer's Disease. http://www.alz.org/national/documents/brochure_endoflifedecisions.pdf.

Alzheimer's Disease International (2016) *World Alzheimer Report 2016. Improving Healthcare for People Living with Dementia; Coverage, Quality and Costs Now and in the Future.* London: Alzheimer's Disease International.

Alzheimer Europe (2008) End-of-Life Care for People with Dementia. http://www.alzheimereurope.org/Ethics/Ethical-issues-in-practice/2008-End-of-Lifecare-for-people-with-dementia.

Amador, S., C. Goodman, D. King, Y.T. Ng et al. (2014) "Exploring resource use and associated costs in end-of-life care for older people with dementia in residential care homes." *International Journal of Geriatric Psychiatry* 29 (7): 758–66.

Araw, M., A. Kozikowski, C. Sison, T. Mir et al. (2015) "Does a palliative care consult decrease the cost of caring for hospitalized patients with dementia?" *Palliative and Supportive Care* 13: 1535–40.

Barak Y. and D. Aizenberg (2002) "Suicide amongst Alzheimer's disease patients: A 10-year survey." *Dementia and Geriatric Cognitive Disorders* 14: 101–03.

de Beaufort, I.D. and S. van de Vathorst (2016) "Dementia and assisted suicide and euthanasia." *Journal of Neurology* 263: 1463–67. https://doi.org/10.1007/s00415-016-8095-2.

Blank, R.H. (1995) *Biomedical Policy*. Chicago: Nelson-Hall.

Blank, R.H. and J. Merrick, eds. (2007) *End-of-Life Decision Making: A Cross-National Study*. Cambridge: MIT Press.

Cohen, S., C. Sprung, P. Sjokvist, A. Lippert et al. (2005) "Communication of end-of-life decisions in European intensive care units." *Intensive Care Medicine* 31 (9): 1215–21

Cox, C.L., E. Cole, T. Reynolds, M. Wandrag et al. (2006) "Implications of cultural diversity in do not attempt resuscitation (DNAR) decisions." *Journal of Multicultural Nursing & Health* 12 (1): 20–28.

Davies, N., L. Maio, G. Rait and S. Iliffe (2014) "Quality end-of-life care for dementia: What have family carers told us so far? A narrative synthesis." *Palliative Medicine* 28: 919–30.

Draper, B., C. Peisaha, J. Snowdond and H. Brodaty (2010) "Early dementia diagnosis and the risk of suicide and euthanasia." *Alzheimer's and Dementia* 6: 75–82.

Dunn, H. (2009) *Hard Choices for Loving People*, 5th ed. Lansdowne, VA: A&A Publishers.

Guidry, M. (2014) "On the boundaries of bioethics: Alzheimer's, dementia, and euthanasia." *Applied Sentience*. https://appliedsentience.com/2014/12/19/on-the-boundaries-of-bioethics-alzheimers-dementia-and-euthanasia/.

Hendriks, S.A., M. Smalbrugge, C.M.P.M. Hertogh and J.T. van der Steen (2014) "Dying with dementia: Symptoms, treatment, and quality of life in the last week of life." *Journal of Pain and Symptom Management* 47 (4): 710–20.

Hertogh, C.M.P.M. (2005) "End-of-life care and medical decision making in patients with dementia." In A. Burns, ed., *Standards in Dementia Care: European Dementia Consensus Network (EDCON)*. New York: Taylor & Francis, pp. 339–54.

Heyman, J.C. and I.A. Gutheil (2010) "Older Latinos' attitudes toward and comfort with end-of-life planning." *Health and Social Work* 35 (1): 17–25.

Humphry, D. (2014) "Can an Alzheimer's victim end their own life?" *Assisted-Dying Blog*. http://assisteddying.org/blog/2011/01/10/can-an-alzheimers-victim-end-their-own-life/.

Johnstone, M-J. (2013) *Alzheimer's Disease, Media Representations and the Politics of Euthanasia: Constructing Risk and Selling Death in an Ageing Society.* Surrey, UK: Ashgate.

Kelley, A.S., N.S. Wenger and C.A. Sarkisian (2010) "Opinions: End-of-life care preferences and planning of older Latinos." *Journal of the American Geriatrics Society* 58 (6): 1109–16.

Kouwenhoven, P.S.C., N.J.H. Raijmakers, J.J.M. van Delden, J.A.C. Rietjens et al. (2015) "Opinions about euthanasia and advanced dementia: A qualitative study among Dutch physicians and members of the general public." *BMC Medical Ethics* 16: 7. http://www.biomedcentral.com/1472-6939/16/7.

Lichtner, V., D. Dowding, P. Esterhuizen, S. José Closs et al. (2014) "Pain assessment for people with dementia: A systematic review of systematic reviews of pain assessment tools." *BMC Geriatrics* 14: 138.

Liu, Y., J.T Yu, H.F. Wang, P.R. Han et al. (2015) "APOE genotype and neuroimaging markers of Alzheimer's disease: Systematic review and meta-analysis." *Journal of Neurology and Neurosurgery Psychiatry* 86 (2): 127–34.

Livingston, G., A. Sommerlad, V. Orgeta, S.G. Costafreda et al. (2017) "Dementia prevention, intervention, and care." *The Lancet.* https://doi.org/10.1016/S0140-6736(17)31363-6.

McCrae, N. (2014) "Assisted suicide and dementia." http://www.carenotkilling.org.uk/medical-opinion/assisted-suicide-and-dementia/.

McCrae, N. and J. Bloomfield (2013) "Mental health nursing and assisted dying." *Journal of Psychiatric & Mental Health Nursing* 20: 655–61.

Miller, F.G. and P.S. Appelbaum (2018) "Physician-assisted death for psychiatric patients—Misguided public policy." *New England Journal of Medicine* 378: 883–85.

Miller, D.G., R. Dresser and S.Y.H. Kim (2018) "Advance euthanasia directives: A controversial case and its ethical implications." *Journal of Medical Ethics.* https://doi.org/10.1136/medethics-2017-104644.

Owen, J.E., K.T. Goode and W.E. Haley (2001) "End of life care and reactions to death in African-American and white family caregivers of relatives with Alzheimer's disease." *Omega (Westport)* 43: 349–61.

Pinzon, L.C.E., M. Claus, K.M. Perrar, K.I. Zepf et al. (2013) "Dying with dementia: Symptom burden, quality of care, and place of death." *Deutsches Ärzteblatt International* 110: 195–202.

Prosporo, S. (2015) "A patient's decision: Dementia and euthanasia." https://sozoprosporo.com/2015/12/.

Rabins, P.V. (2007) "Can suicide be a rational and ethical act in persons with early or pre-dementia?" *American Journal of Bioethics* 7: 47–49.

Sampson, E.L. (2010) "Palliative care for people with dementia." *British Medical Bulletin* 96: 159–74.

Searight, H.R. and J. Gafford (2005) "Cultural diversity at the end of life: Issues and guidelines for family physicians." *American Family Physician* 71 (3): 515–22.

Shrank, W.H., J.S. Kutner, T. Richardson, R.A. Mularski et al. (2005) "Focus group findings about the influences of communication preferences in end-of-life care." *Journal of General Internal Medicine* 2(8): 703–9.

Smith, W.J. (2013) "Swiss suicide clinic kills Alzheimer's patient, euthanasia activists applaud." http://www.lifenews.com/2013/06/09/swiss-suicide-clinic-kills-alzheimers-patient-euthanasia-activists-applaud/

Sprung, C.L., P. Maia, H-H. Bulow, B. Ricou et al. (2007) "The importance of religious affiliation and culture on end-of-life decisions in European intensive care units." *Intensive Care Medicine* 33 (10): 1732–39.

Tomlinson, E. and J. Stott (2014) "Assisted dying in dementia: A systematic review of the international literature on the attitudes of health professionals, patients, carers and the public, and the factors associated with these." *International Journal of Geriatric Psychiatry* 30 (1): 10–20.

van der Steen, J.T. (2010) "Dying with dementia: What we know after more than a decade of research." *Journal of Alzheimer's Disease* 22: 37–55.

van der Steen, J.T., I. Meuleman-Peperkamp and M.W. Ribbe (2009) "Trends in treatment of pneumonia among Dutch nursing home patients with dementia." *Journal of Palliative Medicine* 12: 789–95.

Wada, T., H. Imai, E. Fukutomi et al. (2014) "Preferred feeding methods for dysphagia due to end-stage dementia in community-dwelling elderly people in Japan." *Journal of the American Geriatric Society* 62: 1810–11.

CHAPTER 7

Alzheimer's Policy: Future Directions

Abstract The concluding chapter first recapitulates why policy issues surrounding AD and other dementias are becoming increasingly difficult. It also discusses the issue of rationing medical care by age, which is especially important for AD, and the notion of the technological fix. It then examines the various technological scenarios and the implications of each for AD policy. It concludes by calling for more cross-national political learning in framing anticipatory policies best able to deal with the issues AD raises for society.

Keywords Rationing medical care · Technological fix · Anticipatory policies

All governments make decisions that set priorities regarding regulation and distribution of public goods, and AD is no exception. AD, along with other dementias, is a costly disease that is consuming mounting resources especially from Medicare and Medicaid and from families. It is a global problem, especially hard on low- and middle-income countries (LMICs) which are least able to deal with it and national health services that function under global budgets where money for AD must come from other areas. The great fear and anxiety AD engenders has led to an expanding industry that poses a danger of exploiting those fears through aggressive

R. H. Blank, *Social & Public Policy of Alzheimer's Disease in the United States*, https://doi.org/10.1007/978-981-13-0656-3_7

marketing of brain intervention products, particularly via the Internet, that overpromise and create false hope. This raises question of what, if anything, can governments do to protect highly susceptible citizens from an industry exploiting, and in the process, aggrandizing these fears. Finally, AD policies vary widely across countries regarding innovative AD communities, funding of informal caregivers, and assisted suicide/euthanasia laws, among other areas. More cross-national research on AD policy is needed so that we can better understand what policies work best in dealing with the unfolding AD crisis over the coming decades.

Chapter 2 introduced a wide range of policy areas that are relevant to AD. Although some are more pertinent and encompassing than others, they include funding for research and care, long-term services and support, health promotion and prevention, housing and community services such as adult day care and senior centers, workforce policy and support for family carers, and law enforcement and safeguarding AD patients. Navigating any one of these areas is difficult under the best of circumstances, but people with AD raise particularly exigent legal and ethical issues that center on the question of the capacity to make decisions.

THE ISSUE OF COMPETENCE

Medical practitioners, social workers, researchers, and others working with older adults with AD face uncertainties regarding decisional autonomy and competency, the necessity of timely planning for loss of decision making capacity, and potential conflicts of interest (not all family members consider the best interests of the AD patient). Moreover, they must cope with a maze of proxy directives including durable powers of attorney for health care and/or finances, instructional directives, living wills and estate planning or living trusts, and, ultimately, end-of-life issues such as quality of life, abatement of medical care, and PAS, many of which vary from state to state and across countries. Often these issues focus on questions of competency as the disease progresses.

The informed consent principle specifies that, to be legally valid, consent to medical treatment or research participation must be informed, voluntary, and competent. A major problem with AD, as compared to other chronic illnesses, is the question of competency or capacity to make an informed decision. Competency, or capacity, is a theorized condition that cannot be directly observed or measured with precision yet is fundamental in any social setting. Since it is not a unitary concept, one must always ask competency to do what and in what context. Moreover, a person could be judged competent in some domains, but not in others.

- Treatment consent capacity to make medical decisions
- Research consent capacity to participate in clinical studies and research
- Financial capacity to manage financial affairs or conservatorship
- Capacity to live independently and self-guardianship
- Testamentary capacity to change or make a will
- Capacity to operate a motor vehicle
- Capacity to vote or run for office

The line between competency and incompetency can be a subjective one and will change drastically over the course of AD. It typically denotes a clinical status determined by physician who makes a judgment based on patient's functional, cognitive, and behavioral abilities. Although the clinical finding can be evidence of incompetency, it alone does not determine competency status or automatically transfer authority for decision making to another party. Legal competency or incompetency is an official status determined by a judge based on the clinical as well as lay evidence, case and statutory law of the state, broader principles of justice, and other non-clinical factors. A judgment of incompetency alters legal status by removing rights of self-determination for specific matters and requires the transfer of decisional authority to a court-appointed proxy, a guardian, or a conservator. In a court proceeding, the burden of proof lies with the party alleging that the person is incompetent, although the stigma surrounding AD can make objectivity difficult. Therefore, while a diagnosis of AD or cognitive impairment, in itself, does not constitute incompetency, it certainly is a relevant factor. To make that determination, however, one must examine the actual performance of functional abilities that are integral to consent capacity. While competency status can sometimes be restored over time, this is highly improbable with an AD diagnosis.

One possible policy option could be that prior to or soon after being diagnosed with AD while still legally competent, a person could write an advance directive specifying that it should go into effect at the time they are declared incompetent. If they so desired, this could include provisions to abate life-extending interventions including assisted suicide. The guarantee that this would be carried out according to their wishes at the point they are deemed incompetent could relieve the fears that many persons have against losing control of their life and reduce the number of pre-emptive suicides of those diagnosed with AD before they reach the point of no return. To some extent, this is what the Netherlands and a few other jurisdictions are beginning to allow.

RATIONING BY AGE

The older we become, the more health resources we consume. Average per capita expenditure is approximately four times higher for the elderly than the non-elderly, and, more importantly, the rate of increase in such spending for the elderly is nearly three times that of the non-elderly (CDC 2007). The elderly use more acute care, are hospitalized about twice as often, stay longer in hospitals, and are much more likely to be readmitted to a hospital. In the United States, nearly half of all ICU patients are over age 65, and the cost of ICU care for a patient over age 65 is three to five times more per day than the cost of resources utilized for the average acute-care admission.

Ironically, because of medical improvements and technologies that prolong life, chronic disease requiring frequent medical care has become an ever-increasing drain on medical resources. People who in earlier times would have died of one illness are often kept alive to suffer long-term decline in quality of life, often with AD and/or other chronic conditions (see Box 7.1). Furthermore, because of the concurrence of multiple and often chronic conditions, the cost of prolonging life at older ages is higher than at younger ones, increasingly so since the introduction of antibiotics has reduced the incidence of death from illnesses such as pneumonia.

Box 7.1 Keeping Elderly Alive but at What Cost?
The cost of caring for aging US citizens by 2030 will add 25 percent to the nation's overall health care costs. Even if improved lifestyles and medical technologies reduce the major causes of premature death, we will be left with a growing elderly population whose additional years of life may be dominated by non-fatal, but highly debilitating, conditions such as arthritis, osteoporosis, COPD, and AD. The result could be longer life but worsening health, thus an actual decline in active life expectancy. Under these circumstances, health care becomes Sisyphean, where we conquer one disease only to throw ourselves into the arms of another as we attempt to fill this fiscal black hole by using resources that are desperately needed by other generations (Lamm and Blank 2007).

This disproportionate use of health care resources by the elderly, especially those over age 85, raises the highly provocative issue of rationing that could deny them needed medical technologies (Reese et al. 2010). The most common argument against considering age in making medical decisions is that it is clear age discrimination and patently unfair because of their past contributions to society. Simply put, society owes the elderly their "just rewards." Critics of such rationing also reject economic claims of savings from the denial of care to the elderly on grounds that they are less productive to society or that more disability-adjusted-life-years are gained by giving preference to younger people. Moreover, opponents contest the view that elderly patients are less able to benefit from treatment and reject chronological age as a useful gauge of benefit, arguing that all patients should be assessed for treatment equally based on their physiology alone (Churchill 2005).

In contrast, the "fair innings" argument maintains that it is fitting and just that those who have already received more than their fair share of life defer to the younger generation that has not. Williams (2000) suggests that age should be a criterion in the prioritization of scarce resources, because the alternative is too outrageous to contemplate, namely, that we expect the young to make large sacrifices so that the elderly can enjoy small benefits. Similarly, Callahan (1990) argues that even with relatively ample resources, there are better ways to spend our money than on indefinitely extending the life of a person beyond the "natural lifespan." For Callahan, a natural life span is one in which life's possibilities have largely been achieved and after which death may be understood as a sad, but, nonetheless, reasonably acceptable event. To that end, we should abandon the notion of trying endlessly through medical progress to conquer old age and instead accept aging as a part of life, not just another medical obstacle to overcome.

The debate will persist, but with the aging of the baby boomers, unless something is done to change the skewed spending pattern, this burgeoning cohort will consume an inordinate proportion of health care resources. Simply put, health care costs cannot be controlled without using age as a criterion in rationing simply because the elderly are the heaviest users of technologies that increase the costs of medicine. Although the elderly are logical targets for rationing, given their political influence attempts to explicitly ration medical care on grounds of age currently are non-starters in the United States. Interestingly, although widely condemned in the United States, in other countries such as France and Britain old age "is a criterion for rationing health resources and it occurs at all levels of the National Health Service" (Williams 2000: 198).

Whatever one's view on this topic, there is no denying that the aging population, complicated by AD, makes the distribution of health care resources and, in fact, the redistribution of all societal resources progressively difficult. As the prevalence and costs associated with AD escalate and the informal care workforce shrinks forcing Medicaid, and social welfare systems in other countries, to absorb even greater costs of LTC, cost containment pressures will accelerate. Any debate over setting limits to medical technologies and rationing health care must address the intergenerational redistribution of resources as well as the implications of any policy changes for the elderly. Given increasingly scarce resources, the younger working population is likely object to a greater proportion redistributed from them to the elderly and will demand some rationing of resources away from AD patients. In such a context, a diagnosis of AD could take on even more ominous implications.

Technology Fix Mentality

American culture especially is predisposed toward progress through technological means and identifies quality medicine with high-technology medicine. This unrealistic dependence on technology has translated into a potent desire to find quick technological fixes to all manner of human problems. Not surprisingly, the unremitting development of medical technologies has led to sizable increases in health care expenditures. More than any other factor, this proliferation of medical technology explains the growth of health spending in the United States (Skinner et al. 2006). Although not all technological advances lead to added expenditures, the cumulative effect has been to increase the cost due to extensions in the range and intensity of care. Moreover, while curative treatment may be beneficial to individual patients, the marginal gain in terms of length of survival and quality of life is difficult to judge (Lewis and Leeder 2009).

Public expectations have been elevated unrealistically because of a tendency to oversell medical innovation and exaggerate the capacities of medical intervention. Frequently, the initial response of the media, often encouraged by medical spokespersons, is to report innovations as "breakthroughs." Seldom is there an effort to balance these claims with a discussion about their limitations, complexity, and social implications. With few exceptions, the public is not exposed to comprehensive, systematic, and critical analysis of medical developments. This media coverage generally heightens the public's already strong trust in the technological fix and solidifies the view that if society would only put its collective mind and resources to a task, we will beat the disease at hand. By accentuating the positive and sensational aspects of medical research and development, the media creates idealistic expectations about the power of medicine that opens doors for all forms of charlatans. Importantly, the dependence on technological medicine diverts attention and resources from disease prevention, health promotion, and non-medical health strategies.

The technology fix mindset explains why it is politically more expedient to call for increased funding to find a cure to AD, even when to date that goal has been elusive, rather than shift more resources into the more mundane areas of prevention or care. We are driven by the belief that eventually with enough spending we will conquer AD and "win the war" as we did with polio and other diseases. However, at some point there might be breaking point. After several decades of an almost obsessive ritual of making claims that within five years there will be a cure or at least an effective intervention for AD, that outcome remains unfulfilled. Whitehouse (2014) questions how long the assertion that we are close to a cure can maintain its credibility before the public and policy makers become disillusioned with the lack of progress.

FUTURE SCENARIOS FOR THE ALZHEIMER'S POLICY

Lewis Thomas's (1974) classification of medical technologies as non-technology, half-way technology, or definitive (or advanced) technology is useful here. For Thomas, the determining characteristic is the level of understanding of the disease process which underlies the application of medical theory. Non-technology occurs when doctors have no effective therapy for the disease but might be able to provide some service even if it is only counseling or palliation of symptoms. Although this represents much of early medical practice, it still applies to the management of AD and other degenerative diseases of old age. At the other end, definitive technology for Thomas is not the conventional one of the methods using the most expensive equipment and skills directly on the patient. Instead, it comprises those technologies used when science has a good understanding of the disease process and has developed a specific therapy to counteract it. Definitive medical technologies, then, can be quite simple to administer, for example, a pill or an injection, but they are capable of either preventing a disease (e.g., immunizations) or offering a genuine cure.

In contrast, half-way technologies are not grounded on a thorough comprehension of the biological processes causing the disease, thus, they can neither prevent nor cure disease. While they might in some way compensate for the disease's effect on the patient, they often serve merely to postpone death or to prolong life, but usually with reduced quality. Because of limited knowledge and capacities, half-way interventions are often costly and might divert resources from basic research that could lead to definitive technologies or to preventive strategies. Even if effective drugs are developed for AD, they might keep people out of nursing homes longer, but not diminish the number of older people with cognitive impairment. If such drugs lengthen life, they could increase health care costs and might even cause individuals to live longer with dementia rather than the envisaged goal of improving cognition and averting it.

There are, then, several possible future scenarios that might be considered that will significantly influence AD policy making in the coming decades. The first would be that a definitive prevention or cure for AD is discovered and war on AD is won through medicine. Although this would be game changing, from what has been accomplished thus far, it is most unlikely at least in near future. When, if ever, this scenario transpires, in addition to various regulatory issues, it will raise serious distributive policy issues as to who gets these likely very expensive drugs or technologies and who pays. On a global scale, it raises questions of their availability in LMICs, not unlike that experienced with AIDS drugs.

A second scenario assumes that half-way treatments are found that moderate symptoms and extend the life of AD patients. The most likely half-way technologies at this point are physical interventions like DBS or stem cell therapy or possible new drug regimes. Although this scenario is yet to occur, it is considerably more likely than the first, but it too raises difficult policy issues. First, it encompasses the same regulatory and distributive considerations that advanced technologies generate. Moreover, unless the half-way technologies improve quality of life with lower levels of disability, simply extending the person's life will not ameliorate LTC costs or the burdens of AD and, in fact, might heighten them.

A third scenario is that we fail to uncover the underlying causes of AD and the status quo non-technology persists with no medical success in treating AD. The state of the art for AD technology at present fits largely into the non-technology category, although one might argue that current drugs could be low-end, half-way technologies. On the one hand, this lack of medical progress could encourage the proliferation of fraudulent enterprises that exploit the fears and anxieties that AD raises. On the other hand, it intensifies the need for developing innovative programs to make AD care more humane and give those diagnosed with AD added legal opportunities to control their lives. Therefore, it shifts emphasis from cognitive health to social health.

A fourth scenario is based upon confirmation that an array of non-medical, preventive approaches can reduce AD prevalence significantly. This new evidence should lead to increased public support and funding for health promotion and prevention strategies. Whether it simultaneous reduces funding for continuing the search for definitive technologies would be a political decision. Moreover, while this would be a welcome development, it would do little to diminish the challenges of AD in the near term since the long lead time of AD means that any potential benefits would accrue only to those several decades in the future.

Learning and Policy Transfer

The bottom line is that whichever of these scenarios turns out to be correct, the dilemmas surrounding Alzheimer's that confront policy makers in all countries are destined to intensify to crisis proportions. The need for well-designed anticipatory policy making is critical at this juncture. Although each of the scenarios poses a different set of policy problems in aging populations, it makes it even more imperative to engage in cross-national research to compare how other counties are dealing with these challenges.

Overall, many European countries and Japan have done a better job of dealing with older populations over the last several decades than the United States. Also, some countries including Japan, Germany, and Taiwan have or are instituting programs to fund universal LTC needed in the future. Although it can be risky to transfer policies that work in one country to another, comparative public policy is useful in expanding policy options and demonstrating the experiences of a wide range of applications (Marmor et al. 2009). Examination of international experiences with AD can illuminate both the difficulties faced by, and the wide range of strategies available to, policy makers. They give us cross-cultural insights as to what works or does not work under an array of institutional and cultural contexts. Given the complexity of AD care, comparative studies can generate the evidence necessary to consider the full range of policy options and, therefore, strengthen policy making.

REFERENCES

Callahan, D. (1990) *What Kind of Life? The Limits of Medical Progress.* New York: Simon and Schuster.

Centers for Disease Control and Prevention (CDC) (2007) *The State of Aging and Health in America.* Atlanta, GA: Centers for Disease Control and Prevention.

Churchill, L.R. (2005) "Age-rationing in health care: Flawed policy, personal virtue." *Health Care Analysis* 13 (2): 137–46.

Lamm, R.D. and R.H. Blank (2007) *Condition Critical: A New Moral Vision for U.S. Health Care.* Golden, CO: Fulcrum Press.

Lewis, S.J. and S.R. Leeder (2009) "Why health reform?" *Medical Journal of Australia* 191 (5): 270–72.

Marmor, T.R., R. Freeman and K.G.H. Okma (2009) "Comparative policy analysis and health care: An introduction." In T.R. Marmor, R. Freeman and K.G.H. Okma, eds., *Comparative Studies and the Politics of Modern Medical Care.* New Haven, CT: Yale University Press.

Reese, P.P., A.L. Caplan, R.D. Bloom, P.L. Abt and J.H. Karlawish (2010) "How should we use age to ration health care? Lessons from the case of kidney transplantation." *Journal of the American Geriatric Society* 58: 1980–86.

Skinner, J.S., D.O. Staiger and E.S. Fisher (2006) "Is technological change in medicine always worth it? The case of myocardial infarction." *Health Affairs* 25: w34–w47.

Thomas, L.G. (1974) *The Lives of a Cell.* New York: Viking Press.

Whitehouse, P.J. (2014) "The end of Alzheimer's disease—From biochemical pharmacology to ecopsychosociology: A personal perspective." *Biochemical Pharmacology* 88 (4): 677–81.

Williams, B.O. (2000) "Ageism helps to ration medical treatment." *Health Bulletin* 58 (3): 198–202.

REFERENCES

AARP (2017) Global Council on Brain Health. http://www.aarp.org/health/brain-health/global-council-on-brain-health.

Abou-Saleh, M.T., C. Katona and A. Kumar (2011) *Principles and Practice of Geriatric Psychiatry*, 3rd ed. New York: John Wiley & Sons.

Adaes, S. (2015) "tDCS—A therapy for the future?" http://brainblogger.com/2015/03/05/tcds-a-therapy-for-the-future/.

Ahronheim, J.C., M. Mulvihill, C. Sieger, P. Park and B.E. Fries (2001) "State practice variations in the use of tube feeding for nursing home residents with severe cognitive impairment." *Journal of the American Geriatric Society* 49: 148–52.

Albrecht, J.S., A.L. Gruber-Baldini, E.K. Fromme, J.C. McGregor, D.S. Lee and J.P. Furuno (2013) "Quality of hospice care for individuals with dementia." *Journal of the American Geriatric Society* 61 (7): 1060–5.

Alonso Vilatela, M.E., M. Lopez-Lopez and P. Yescas-Gomez (2012) "Genetics of Alzheimer's Disease." *Archives of Medical Research* 43: e622–e631.

Alper, J. (2006) *The Partnership for Long-term Care: A Public-Private Partnership to Finance Long-term Care*. Robert Wood Johnson Foundation.

Alzheimer's Association (2016a) "Alzheimer's disease facts and figures." *Alzheimer's and Dementia* 12 (4). https://www.alz.org/documents_custom/2016-facts-and-figures.pdf.

Alzheimer's Association (2016b) End-of-life decisions: Honoring the wishes of a person with Alzheimer's Disease. http://www.alz.org/national/documents/brochure_endoflifedecisions.pdf.

Alzheimer's Association (2016c) Alzheimer's Disease State Plans. http://act.alz. org/site/PageNavigator/state_plans.html.

Alzheimer's Association (2016d) Tests for Alzheimer's Disease and Dementia. http://www.alz.org/alzheimers_disease_steps_to_diagnosis.asp.

Alzheimer's Association (2017) "Beta-amyloid and the amyloid hypothesis." https://www.alz.org/documents/national/topicsheet_betaamyloid.pdf.

Alzheimer's Association (2018) "Alzheimer's disease facts and figures." *Alzheimer's and Dementia* 14 (3): 367–429.

Alzheimer's Association and Centers for Disease Control and Prevention (2013) *The Healthy Brain Initiative: The Public Health Road Map for State and National Partnerships, 2013–2018*. Chicago, IL: Alzheimer's Association.

Alzheimer's Disease International (2013) *Policy Brief for Heads of Government: The Global Impact of Dementia 2013–2050*. London: Alzheimer's Disease International.

Alzheimer's Disease International (2016) *World Alzheimer Report 2016. Improving Healthcare for People Living with Dementia; Coverage, Quality and Costs Now and in the Future*. London: Alzheimer's Disease International.

Alzheimer Europe (2008) End-of-Life Care for People with Dementia. http://www.alzheimereurope.org/Ethics/Ethical-issues-in-practice/2008-End-of-Lifecare-for-people-with-dementia.

Alzheimer Europe (2016) National Dementia Strategies. http://alzheimer-europe.org/Policy-in-Practice2/National-Dementia-Strategies/.

Alzheimer's Impact Movement (2018) "BOLD Infrastructure for Alzheimer's Act." https://alzimpact.org/priorities/bold_alzheimers_act?WT.mc_id=enews2018_04_04&utm_source=enews-aff-38&utm_medium=email&utm_campaign=enews-2018-04-04.

Alzheimer's News (2018) "Congress prioritizes Alzheimer's and dementia research funding in 2018 budget." https://alz.org/news_and_events_105707.asp?WT.mc_id=enews2018_03_21&utm_source=enews-aff-38&utm_medium=email&utm_campaign=enews-2018-03-21.

Amador, S., C. Goodman, D. King, Y.T. Ng et al. (2014) "Exploring resource use and associated costs in end-of-life care for older people with dementia in residential care homes." *International Journal of Geriatric Psychiatry* 29 (7): 758–66.

Ampe, S., A. Sevenants, E. Coppens, N. Spruytte et al. (2015) "Study protocol for 'we DECide': Implementation of advance care planning for nursing home residents with dementia. *Journal of Advanced Nursing* 71 (5): 1156–62.

Araw, M., A. Kozikowski, C. Sison, T. Mir et al. (2015) "Does a palliative care consult decrease the cost of caring for hospitalized patients with dementia?" *Palliative and Supportive Care* 13: 1535–40.

Ardekani, B.A., A. Convit and A.H. Bachman (2016) "Analysis of the MIRIAS data shows sex differences in hippocampal atrophy progression." *Journal of Alzheimer's Disease* 50: 3.

Ausserhofer, D., M. Deschodt and S. De Geest (2016) "There's no place like home: A scoping review on the impact of homelike residential care models on resident-, family-, and staff-related outcomes." *Journal of American Medical Directors Association* 17: 685–93.

Ballard, C., A. Corbett and R. Howard (2014) "Prescription of antipsychotics in people with dementia." *British Journal of Psychiatry* 205: 4–5.

Ballard, C.A., M. Orrell, S. YongZhong, E. Moniz-Cook et al. (2016) "Impact of antipsychotic review and nonpharmacological intervention on antipsychotic use, neuropsychiatric symptoms, and mortality in people with dementia living in nursing homes: A factorial cluster randomized controlled trial by the Well-Being and Health for People with Dementia (WHELD) program." *American Journal of Psychiatry* 173: 252–62.

Barak Y. and D. Aizenberg (2002) "Suicide amongst Alzheimer's disease patients: A 10-year survey." *Dementia and Geriatric Cognitive Disorders* 14: 101–03.

Barnes, D.E. and K. Yaffe (2011) "The projected effect of risk factor reduction on Alzheimer's disease prevalence." *The Lancet Neurology* 10 (9): 819–28.

Bartus, R.T., R.L. Dean III, B. Beer and A.S. Lippa (1982) "The cholinergic hypothesis of geriatric memory dysfunction." *Science* 217: 408–14.

Basting, A.D. (2009) *Forget Memory: Creating Better Lives for People with Dementia*. Boston: Johns Hopkins Press.

Baum, M.L. (2016) "Patient requests for off-label bioprediction of dementia." *Clinical Neuroethics* 25 (4): 686–90. https://doi.org/10.1017/S0963180116000402.

Baumgart, M., H.M. Snyder, M.C. Carrillo, S. Fazio et al. (2015) "Summary of the evidence on modifiable risk factors for cognitive decline and dementia: A population-based perspective." *Alzheimer's & Dementia: The Journal of the Alzheimer's Association* 11 (6): 718–26.

BCBS (2016) "Corporate medical policy: Genetic testing for Alzheimer's disease." https://www.bcbsnc.com/assets/services/public/pdfs/medicalpolicy/genetic_testing_for_alzheimers_disease.pdf.

de Beaufort, I.D. and S. van de Vathorst (2016) "Dementia and assisted suicide and euthanasia." *Journal of Neurology* 263: 1463–67. https://doi.org/10.1007/s00415-016-8095-2.

Beerens, H.C., S.M. Zwakhalen, H. Verbeek, D. Ruwaard and J.P. Hamers (2013) "Factors associated with quality of life of people with dementia in long-term care facilities: A systematic review." *International Journal of Nursing Studies* 50: 1259–70.

Bellamy, J. (2015) "Society for Science-Based Medicine: Comment to FDA on homeopathic drug regulation." https://sciencebasedmedicine.org/society-for-science-based-medicine-comment-to-fda-on-homeopathic-drug-regulation/.

Bernier, P.J., C. Gourdeau, P-H. Carmichael, J-P. Beauchemin et al. (2017) "Validation and diagnostic accuracy of predictive curves for age-associated longitudinal cognitive decline in older adults." *Canadian Medical Association Journal* 189: E1472–E1480.

Bjelakovic, G., D. Nikolova, L.L. Gluud, R.G. Simonetti and C. Gluud (2012) "Antioxidant supplements for prevention of mortality in healthy participants and patients with various diseases." *Cochrane Database Systems Review* 14 (3): CD007176. https://doi.org/10.1002/14651858.CD007176.pub2.

Blank, R.H. (1995) *Biomedical Policy*. Chicago: Nelson-Hall.

Blank, R.H. (2015) *Cognitive Enhancement: Social and Public Policy Issues*. London: Palgrave Press.

Blank, R.H. and J. Merrick, eds. (2007) *End-of-Life Decision Making: A Cross-National Study*. Cambridge: MIT Press.

Boggio, P.S., L.P. Khoury, D.C. Martins, O.E. Martins et al. (2009) "Temporal cortex direct current stimulation enhances performance on a visual recognition memory task in Alzheimer disease." *Journal of Neurology and Neurosurgery Psychiatry* 80 (4): 444–47.

Boot, W.R. and A.F. Kramer (2014) "The brain-games conundrum: Does cognitive training really sharpen the mind?" Cerebrum. http://dana.org/Cerebrum/2014/The_Brain-ames_Conundrum__Does_Cognitive_Training_Really_Sharpen_the_Mind_/.

Boots, L.M.M., M.E. Vugt, R.J.M. Knippenberg et al. (2014) "A systematic review of Internet-based supportive interventions for caregivers of patients with dementia." *International Journal of Geriatric Psychiatry* 29 (4): 331–44.

Borenstein, A. and J. Mortimer (2016) *Alzheimer's Disease: Life Course Perspectives on Risk Reduction*. Cambridge, MA: Academic Press.

Bowler, J.V. and V. Hachinski, eds. (2003) *Vascular Cognitive Impairment: Preventable Dementia*. Oxford: Oxford University Press.

Bredesen, D.E. (2014) "Reversal of cognitive decline: A novel therapeutic program." *Aging* 6 (9): 707–17.

Bredesen, D.E., E.C. Amos, J. Canick, M. Ackerley et al. (2016) "Reversal of cognitive decline in Alzheimer's disease." *Aging* 8 (6): 1250–58.

Brier, M.R., B. Gordon, K. Friedrichsen, J. McCarthy et al. (2016) "Tau and Ab imaging, CSF measures, and cognition in Alzheimer's disease." *Science Translational Medicine* 3 (338): 338ra66.

Burau, V., H. Theobald and R.H. Blank (2007) *Governing Home Care: A Cross-National Comparison*. London: Edward Elgar.

Burns, A. and P. Robert (2009) "The national dementia strategy in England." *British Medical Journal* 338: b931.

Burstein, A.A., O. DaDalt, B. Kramer, L. D'Ambrosio and J. Coughlin (2014) "Technology and the caregiving dilemma: A comparative look at awareness, attitudes, and the role of technology." *Alzheimer's and Dementia* 10 (Suppl): 571.

Bynum, J.P.W. (2014) "The long reach of Alzheimer's disease: Patients, practice, and policy." *Health Affairs* 33 (4): 534–40.

Callahan, D. (1990) *What Kind of Life? The Limits of Medical Progress.* New York: Simon and Schuster.

Campbell, J., N. Ikegami, C. Gori, F. Barbabella et al. (2016) "How different countries allocate long-term care resources to older users: A comparative snapshot." In C. Gori, J-L. Fernández and R. Wittenberg, eds., *Long-term Care Reforms in OECD Countries: Successes and Failures.* Bristol: Policy Press, pp. 47–76.

Centers for Disease Control and Prevention (CDC) (2007) *The State of Aging and Health in America.* Atlanta, GA: Centers for Disease Control and Prevention.

Chan, A.L., T-M. Cham and S-J. Lin (2009) "Direct medical costs in patients with Alzheimer's disease in Taiwan: A population-based study." *Current Therapeutic Research, Clinical and Experimental* 70 (1): 10–18.

Chin, A.L., S. Negash and R. Hamilton (2011) "Diversity and disparity in dementia: The impact of ethnoracial differences in Alzheimer disease." *Alzheimer Disease and Associated Disorders* 25 (3): 187–95.

Chirles, T.J., K. Reiter, L.R. Weiss, A.J. Alfini et al. (2017) "Exercise training and functional connectivity changes in mild cognitive impairment and healthy elders." *Journal of Alzheimer's Disease* 57 (3): 845–56. https://doi.org/10.3233/JAD-161151.

CHKS (2012) "An economic analysis of the excess costs for acute care for patients with dementia." CHKS, 2012. http://www.chks.co.uk/userfiles/files/Dementia_an_economic_analysis.pdf

Cholerton, B., E.B. Larson, L.D. Baker et al. (2013) "Neuropathologic correlates of cognition in a population-based sample." *Journal of Alzheimer's Disease* 36: 699–709

Churchill, L.R. (2005) "Age-rationing in health care: Flawed policy, personal virtue." *Health Care Analysis* 13 (2): 137–46.

Clarfield, A.M. (2003) "The decreasing prevalence of reversible dementias: An up-dated meta-analysis." *Archives of Internal Medicine* 163 (18): 2219–29

Clark, P.C., N.G. Kutner, F.C. Goldstein, S. Peterson-Hazen et al. (2005) "Impediments to timely diagnosis of Alzheimer's disease in African Americans." *Journal of the American Geriatrics Society* 53 (11): 2012–17

Cohen, S., C. Sprung, P. Sjokvist, A. Lippert et al. (2005) "Communication of end-of-life decisions in European intensive care units." *Intensive Care Medicine* 31 (9): 1215–21

Cohen-Mansfield, J., D. Shmotkin and S. Goldberg (2009) "Loneliness in old age: Longitudinal changes and their determinants in an Israeli sample." *International Journal of Psychogeriatrics* 21: 1160–70

Collins, F. (2014) "What to expect in brain health research in 2015." *AARP Bulletin.* http://www.aarp.org/health/brain-health/info-2014/brain-health-research.html?intcmp=AE-HEA-RELBOX.

Commission on Long-Term Care (2013) *A Comprehensive Approach to Long-Term Services and Supports.* Washington, DC: Commission on Long-Term Care

Connelly, K., K. ur Rehman Laghari, M. Mokhtari and T.H. Falk (2014) "Approaches to understanding the impact of technologies for aging in place: A mini-review." *Gerontology* 60: 282–88

Conrad, P. and A. Horwitz (2013) "Marketing of neuropsychiatric illness and enhancement." In A. Chatterjee and M.J. Farah, eds., *Neuroethics in Practice: Medicine, Mind, and Society.* New York: Oxford University Press, pp. 46–56.

Consensus on the Brain Training Industry from the Scientific Community (2014) http://longevity.stanford.edu/a-consensus-on-the-brain-training-industry-from-the-scientific-community-2/.

Cooper, C., A. Selwood, M. Blanchard, Z. Walker et al. (2010) "The determinants of family carers' abusive behaviour to people with dementia: Results of the CARD study." *Journal of Affective Disorders* 121: 136–42

Corbett, A., J. Stevens, D. Aarsland et al. (2012) "Systematic review of services providing information and/or advice to people with dementia and/or their caregivers." *International Journal of Geriatric Psychiatry* 27: 628–36

Corbett, A., A.M. Owen, A. Hampshire, J. Grahn et al. (2015) "The effect of an online cognitive training package in healthy older adults: An online randomized controlled trial." *Journal of the American Medical Directors Association* 16: 990–97.

Cote, D.J., A.L. Bredenoord, T.R. Smith, M. Ammirati et al. (2017) "Ethical clinical translation of stem cell interventions for neurologic disease." *Neurology* 88 (3): 322–28.

Cotelli, M., R. Manenti, M. Brambilla, M. Petesi et al. (2014) "Anodal tDCS during face-name associations memory training in Alzheimer's patients." *Frontiers in Aging Neuroscience.* https://doi.org/10.3389/fnagi.2014.00038

Coveney, C., J. Gabe and S. Williams (2011) "The sociology of cognitive enhancement: Medicalisation and beyond." *Health Sociology Review* 20 (4): 381–93.

Cox, C.L., E. Cole, T. Reynolds, M. Wandrag et al. (2006) "Implications of cultural diversity in do not attempt resuscitation (DNAR) decisions." *Journal of Multicultural Nursing & Health* 12 (1): 20–28.

Cummings, J., G. Lee, T. Mortsdorf, A. Ritter and K. Zhong (2017) "Alzheimer's disease drug development pipeline: 2017." *Alzheimer's & Dementia: Translational Research & Clinical Interventions* 3 (3): 367–84.

Dalton, A.M., N. Wareham, S. Griffin and A.P. Jones (2016) "Neighbourhood greenspace is associated with a slower decline in physical activity in older adults: A prospective cohort study." *SSM—Population Health* 2: 683–91.

Dam, A.E., M.E. de Vugt, I.P. Klinkenberg, F.R. Verhey, and M.P. van Boxtel (2016) "A systematic review of social support interventions for caregivers of people with dementia: Are they doing what they promise?" *Maturitas* 85: 117–30.

Davies, N., L. Maio, G. Rait and S. Iliffe (2014) "Quality end-of-life care for dementia: What have family carers told us so far? A narrative synthesis." *Palliative Medicine* 28: 919–30.

de Boer, M.E., C.M.P.M. Hertogh, R. Droes et al. (2007) "Suffering from dementia: The patient's perspective." *International Psychogeriatrics* 19 (6): 1021–39.

de Boer, M.E., R-M. Dröes, C. Jonker, J.A. Eefsting and M.P.M. Hertogh (2011) "Advance directives for euthanasia in dementia: How do they affect resident care in Dutch nursing homes? Experiences of physicians and relatives." *Journal of American Geriatrics Society* 59 (6): 989–96.

de Jager, C.A., A. Oulhaj, R. Jacoby, H. Refsum and A.D. Smith (2012) "Cognitive and clinical outcomes of homocysteine-lowering B-vitamin treatment in mild cognitive impairment: A randomized controlled trial." *International Journal of Geriatric Psychiatry* 27: 592–600.

Department of Health (2013) *Dementia: A State of the Nation Report on Dementia Care and Support in England.* London: Department of Health.

Department of Health and Human Services (DHHS) (2014) National Alzheimer's Project Act. http://aspe.hhs.gov/daltcp/napa/.

Department of Health and Human Services (DHHS) (2016) National Plan to Address Alzheimer's Disease: 2016 Update. https://aspe.hhs.gov/report/national-plan-address-alzheimers-disease-2016-update

Diehl-Schmid, J., R. Jox, S. Gauthier and S. Belleville (2017) "Suicide and assisted dying in dementia: What we know and what we need to know. A narrative literature review." *International Psychogeriatrics.* https://doi.org/10.1017/S1041610217000679.

Dong X., R. Chen and M.A. Simon (2014) "Elder abuse and dementia: A review of the research and health policy." *Health Affairs* 33 (4): 642–49.

Dotinga, R. (2014) "Brain stimulation shows promise against Alzheimer's." http://www.webmd.com/alzheimers/news/20140506/brain-stimulation-shows-early-promise-against-alzheimers#1.

Doty, P. (2010) "The evolving balance of formal and informal, institutional and non-institutional long-term care for older Americans: A thirty-year perspective." *Public Policy and Aging Report* 20 (1): 3–9.

Drakos, A. (2015) "tDCS and Alzheimer's Disease." *Brainstorm Blog.* http://www.tdcsbrainstorm.com/brainstormblog/tdcs-and-alzheimers-disease.

Draper, B., C. Peisaha, J. Snowdond and H. Brodaty (2010) "Early dementia diagnosis and the risk of suicide and euthanasia." *Alzheimer's and Dementia* 6: 75–82.

Dröes, R.M., R. Chattat, A. Diaz, D. Gove et al. (2017) "Social health and dementia: A European consensus on the operationalization of the concept and directions for research and practice." *Aging and Mental Health* 21 (1): 4–17.

Dunn, H. (2009) *Hard Choices for Loving People*, 5th ed. Lansdowne, VA: A&A Publishers.

Duthey, B. (2013) "Alzheimer disease and other dementias." Background Paper 6.11. http://www.who.int/medicines/areas/priority_medicines/BP6_11Alzheimer. pdf.

Dysken, M.W., M. Sano, S. Asthana, J.E. Vertrees et al. (2014) "Effect of vitamin E and memantine on functional decline in Alzheimer disease: The TEAM-AD VA cooperative randomized trial." *Journal of the American Medical Association* 311: 33–44.

Eisenberg, R. (2017) "The troubling AARP long-term care scorecard." *Forbes.* https://www.forbes.com/sites/nextavenue/2017/06/14/the-troubling-aarp-long-term-care-scorecard/#2c7fccde6b25.

Elder, G.J. and J-P. Taylor (2014) "Transcranial magnetic stimulation and transcranial direct current stimulation: Treatments for cognitive and neuropsychiatric symptoms in the neurodegenerative dementias?" *Alzheimer's Research and Therapy* 6: 74–85.

Feinberg, L., S.C. Reinhard, A. Houser and R. Choula (2011) *Valuing the Invaluable: 2011 Update: The Growing Contributions and Costs of Family Caregiving.* Washington, DC: AARP Public Policy Institute.

Ferrucci, R., F. Mameli, I. Guidi, S. Mrakic-Sposta et al. (2008) "Transcranial direct current stimulation improves recognition memory in Alzheimer disease." *Neurology* 71 (7): 493–98.

"First euthanasia in Netherlands of severe Alzheimer's patient performed." Agence France-Presse | November 9, 2011. A National Platform for the Next Generation of Humanist Thinkers.

"First UK assisted suicide for dementia" (2013) http://www.bbc.com/news/health-22715363.

Fleming, R. and N. Purandare (2010) "Long-term care for people with dementia: Environmental design guidelines." *International Psychogeriatrics* 22 (7): 1084–96.

Fleming, R. and S. Sum (2014) "Empirical studies on the effectiveness of assistive technology in the care of people with dementia: A systematic review." *Journal of Assistive Technologies* 8 (1): 14–34.

Forlini, C. and W. Hall (2017) "A prospectus for ethical analysis of ageing individuals' responsibility to prevent cognitive decline." *Bioethics.* https://doi.org/10.1111/bioe.12387.

Francis, P.T., A.M. Palmer, M. Snape and G.K. Wilcock (1999) "The cholinergic hypothesis of Alzheimer's disease: A review of progress." *Journal of Neurology, Neurosurgery, and Psychiatry* 66: 137–47.

Frankish, H. and R. Horton (2017) "Prevention and management of dementia: A priority for public health." *The Lancet.* https://doi.org/10.1016/S0140-6736(17)31756-7.

Frisoni, G.B., M. Boccardi, F. Barkhof, K. Blennow et al. (2017) "Strategic roadmap for an early diagnosis of Alzheimer's disease based on biomarkers." *The Lancet* 16 (8): 661–76.

Fuh, J-L. and S-J. Wang (2008) "Dementia in Taiwan: Past, present, and future." *Acta Neurologica Taiwanica* 17 (1): 153–61.

Fukui, T. (2016) "Disentangling dementia from neuropsychological perspectives." *Japanese Journal of Neuropsychology* 32 (3): 229–38.

Gallagher, D., A. Ni Mhaolain, L. Crosby et al. (2013) "Determinants of the desire to institutionalize in Alzheimer's caregivers." *American Journal of Alzheimer's Disease and Other Dementias* 26: 205–11.

Garrett, M.D. (2013) "Fear of dementia: The emerging fear in America." *Psychology Today.* https://www.psychologytoday.com/blog/iage/201305/fear-dementia.

Geldmacher D.S., N.Y. Kirson, H.G. Birnbaum, S. Eapen et al. (2013) "Pre-diagnosis excess acute care costs in Alzheimer's patients among a U.S. Medicaid population." *Applied Health Economics and Health Policy* 11 (4): 407–13.

Genova, L. (2008) "Busting the myth of Alzheimer's." http://lisagenova.com/busting-the-myth-of-alzheimers-2/.

Ghoravshi, A. (2014) "Brain games exploit anxieties about memory loss for profit." *The Guardian.* http://www.theguardian.com/science/2014/oct/23/brain-games-memory-loss-open-letter#sthash.CSyjdlU2.dpuf.

Giebel, C.M., D. Challisand and D. Montaldi (2015) "Understanding the cognitive underpinnings of functional impairments in early dementia: A review." *Aging and Mental Health* 19 (10): 859–75.

Gilbert, F. and D. Ovadia (2011) "Deep brain stimulation in the media: Over-optimistic portrayals call for a new strategy involving journalists and scientists in ethical debates." *Frontiers in Integrative Neuroscience* 5: 16. https://doi.org/10.3389/fnint.2011.00016.

Gitlin, L.N., L. Winter and M. Dennis (2010) "Assistive devices caregivers use and find helpful to manage problem behaviors of dementia." *Gerontechnology* 9 (3): 408–14.

Gitlin, L.N., W.W. Hauck, M.P. Dennis, L. Winter et al. (2009) "Long-term effect on mortality of a home intervention that reduces functional difficulties in older adults: Results from a randomized trial." *Journal of the American Geriatrics Society* 57 (3): 476–81.

Gordon, M. (2015) "Alzheimer's disease, media representations and the politics of euthanasia: Constructing risk and selling death in an ageing society by Megan-Jane Johnstone (review)." *Canadian Journal on Aging/La Revue canadienne du vieillissement* 34 (2): 258–60.

Goren, A., W. Montgomery, K. Kahle-Wrobleski, T. Nakamura and K. Ueda (2016) "Impact of caring for persons with Alzheimer's disease or dementia on caregivers' health outcomes: Findings from a community based survey in Japan." *BMC Geriatrics* 16: 122.

Greaves, I. and D. Jolly (2010) "National dementia strategy: Well intentioned, but how well founded and how well directed?" *British Journal of General Practice* 60 (572): 193–98.

G-Science Academiers (2016) "G-Science Academies statement 2016: Understanding, protecting, and developing global brain resources." http:// fpcj.jp/wp/wp-content/uploads/2016/05/3Three-Joint-Statements-of-G-Science-Academies-2016.pdf.

Guidry, M. (2014) "On the boundaries of bioethics: Alzheimer's, dementia, and euthanasia." *Applied Sentience*. https://appliedsentience.com/2014/12/19/on-the-boundaries-of-bioethics-alzheimers-dementia-and-euthanasia/.

Gullettemay, M.M. (2011) "Our irrational fear of forgetting." *New York Times*. http://www.nytimes.com/2011/05/22/opinion/22gullette.html.

Hanrahan, D. (2013) "Ethical issues surrounding direct-to-consumer advertising of neurotechnology." *Ethics in Biology, Engineering and Medicine: An International Journal*: 173–84. https://doi.org/10.1615/Ethics BiologyEngMed.2013007012.

Harvard Stem Cell Institute (2016) http://hsci.harvard.edu/alzheimers-disease-0.

Hayden, E.C. (2008) "Alzheimer's tests under fire." *Nature* 455: 30.

Hedman, A., L. Nygård, O. Almkvist and A. Kottorp (2015) "Amount and type of everyday technology use over time in older adults with cognitive impairment." *Scandinavian Journal of Occupational Therapy* 22 (3): 196–206.

Henderson, S.T., J.L. Vogel, L.J. Barr, F. Garvin et al. (2009) "Study of the ketogenic agent AC-1202 in mild to moderate Alzheimer's disease: A randomized, double-blind, placebo-controlled, multicenter trial." *Nutrition and Metabolism* 6: 31.

Hendriks, S.A., M. Smalbrugge, C.M.P.M. Hertogh and J.T. van der Steen (2014) "Dying with dementia: Symptoms, treatment, and quality of life in the last week of life." *Journal of Pain and Symptom Management* 47 (4): 710–20.

Hertogh, C.M.P.M. (2005) "End-of-life care and medical decision making in patients with dementia." In A. Burns, ed., *Standards in Dementia Care: European Dementia Consensus Network (EDCON)*. New York: Taylor & Francis, pp. 339–54.

Heyman, J.C. and I.A. Gutheil (2010) "Older Latinos' attitudes toward and comfort with end-of-life planning." *Health and Social Work* 35 (1): 17–25.

Hodgson, L.J. (2011) "Strategizing about Alzheimer's." *The Gerontologist* 51 (6): 876–80.

Hoffman, D. (2015) "Looking at the future of Alzheimer's disease policy." *Health Affairs Health Policy Lab*. http://healthaffairs.org/blog/2015/07/14/looking-at-the-future-of-alzheimers-disease-policy/.

Hohenfeld, C., N. Nellessen, I. Dogan, H. Kuhn et al. (2017) "Cognitive improvement and brain changes after real-time functional MRI: Neurofeedback training in healthy elderly and prodromal Alzheimer's disease." *Frontiers in Neurology* 8: 384. https://doi.org/10.3389/fneur.2017.00384.

Honig, L.S., B. Vellas, M. Woodward, M. Boada et al. (2018) "Trial of solanezumab for mild dementia due to Alzheimer's disease." *New England Journal of Medicine* 378 (4): 321–30.

Hörder, H., L. Johansson, X-X. Guo and G. Grimby (2018) "Midlife cardiovascular fitness and dementia A 44-year longitudinal population study in women." *Neurology.* https://doi.org/10.1212/WNL.0000000000005290.

Houser, A., M.J. Gibson and D. Redfoot (2010) "Trends in family caregiving and paid home care for older people with disabilities in the community." Washington, DC: AARP Public Policy Institute.

Howard, R. (2005) "Vascular cognitive impairment: Preventable dementia." *American Journal of Psychiatry* 162 (1): 199–200.

Hsieh, E. (2015) "On the horizon: A magnetic zap that strengthens memory." *Scientific American Mind* 26 (3): 15. https://doi.org/10.1038/scientificamericanmind0515-15a.

Huber, M., J.A. Knottnerus, L. Green and H. van der Horst (2011) "How should we define health?" *British Medical Journal* 343: d4163.

Humphry, D. (2014) "Can an Alzheimer's victim end their own life?" *Assisted-Dying Blog.* http://assisteddying.org/blog/2011/01/10/can-an-alzheimers-victim-end-their-own-life/.

Humphreys, G. (2009) "Direct-to-consumer advertising under fire." *Bulletin of the World Health Organization* 87: 576–77.

Hung, Y-N., K. Zbigniew, A.J.M. Brnabic, J-F. Yeh et al. (2016) "The epidemiology and burden of Alzheimer's disease in Taiwan utilizing data from the National Health Insurance Research Database." *ClinicoEconomics and Outcomes Research* 8. https://doi.org/10.2147/CEOR.S93323.

Huntley, J.D., R.L. Gould, K. Liu, M. Smith and R.J. Howard (2015) "Do cognitive interventions improve general cognition in dementia? A meta-analysis and meta-regression." *BMJ Open* 5: e005247.

Hurd, M.D., P. Martorell, A. Delavande, K.J. Mullen and K.M. Langa (2013) "Monetary costs of dementia in the United States." *New England Journal of Medicine* 368 (14): 1326–34.

Innes, A. (2002) "The social and political context of formal dementia care provision." *Ageing and Society* 22: 483–99.

Innes, A. (2009) *Dementia Studies: A Social Science Perspective.* London: Sage Publications.

Innes, A. and B. Director (2013) "Working towards dementia friendly societies." *Perspectives in Public Health* 133 (3): 141.

Innes, A. and J. Manthorpe (2013) "Developing theoretical understandings of dementia and their application to dementia care policy in the UK." *Dementia* 12 (6). http://journals.sagepub.com/doi/abs/10.1177/1471301212442583.

IOM (Institute of Medicine) (2015) *Cognitive Aging: Progress in Understanding and Opportunities for Action.* Washington, DC: The National Academies Press.

James, B.D., S.E. Leurgans, L.E. Hebert, P.A. Scherr et al. (2014) "Contribution of Alzheimer's disease to mortality in the United States." *Neurology* 82 (12): 1045–50.

Jaret, P. (2014) "A test for Alzheimer's disease raises thorny ethical issues." *AARP Bulletin* (May). http://www.aarp.org/health/brain-health/info-2014/alzheimers-disease-blood-test.html?intcmp=AE-HEA-RELBOX.

Johnson, R.A. and J. Karlawish (2015) "A review of ethical issues in dementia." *International Psychogeriatric* 27 (10): 1635–47.

Johnston, B., S. Lawton, C. McCaw, E. Law et al. (2016) "Living well with dementia: Enhancing dignity and quality of life, using a novel intervention, dignity therapy." *International Journal of Older People Nursing* 11 (2): 107–20.

Johnstone, M-J. (2013) *Alzheimer's Disease, Media Representations and the Politics of Euthanasia: Constructing Risk and Selling Death in an Ageing Society.* Surrey, UK: Ashgate.

Kane, R.L., M. Butler, H.A. Fink, M. Brasure et al. (2017) "Interventions to prevent age-related cognitive decline, mild cognitive impairment, and clinical Alzheimer's-type dementia." Comparative Effectiveness Review 188. Rockville, MD: Agency for Healthcare Research and Quality.

Kang, J.M., B.K. Yeon, S.J. Cho and Y.H. Suh (2016) "Stem cell therapy for Alzheimer's disease: A review of recent clinical trials." *Journal of Alzheimer's Disease* 54 (3): 879–89.

Keenan, T.A. (2010) "Planning for long-term care: A survey of midlife and older women." AARP Research Report.

Kelley, A.S., N.S. Wenger and C.A. Sarkisian (2010) "Opinions: End-of-life care preferences and planning of older Latinos." *Journal of the American Geriatrics Society* 58 (6): 1109–16.

Kelley, A.S., K. McGarry, R. Gorges and J.S. Skinner (2015) "The burden of health care costs in the last 5 years of life." *Annals of Internal Medicine* 163 (10): 729–36.

Khedr, E.M., N.F. El Gamal, N.A. El-Fetoh et al. (2014) "A double-blind randomized clinical trial on the efficacy of cortical direct current stimulation for the treatment of Alzheimer's disease." *Frontiers in Aging Neuroscience.* https://doi.org/10.3389/fnagi.2014.00275.

Kim, D.H., S.H. Yeo, J.M. Park, J.Y. Choi et al. (2014) "Genetic markers for diagnosis and pathogenesis of Alzheimer's disease." *Gene* 545 (2): 185–93.

Kindell, J., J. Keady, K. Sage and R. Wilkinson (2017) "Everyday conversation in dementia: A review of the literature to inform research and practice." *International Journal of Language and Communicative Disorders* 52 (4): 392–406.

King, J.B., K.G. Jones, E. Goldberg, M. Rollins, K. MacNamee et al. (2018) "Increased functional connectivity after listening to favoured music in adults with Alzheimer dementia." *The Journal of Prevention of Alzheimer's Disease.* https://doi.org/10.14283/jpad.2018.19.

Knapp, M., J. Barlow, A. Comras-Herrera et al. (2015) "The case for investment in technology to manage the global costs of dementia." http://eprints.lse.ac.uk/66482/1/__lse.ac.uk_storage_LIBRARY_Secondary_libfile_shared_ repository_Content_LSEE_The%20case%20for%20investment%20in%20 technology.

Knapton, S. (2014) "Alzheimer's disease could be prevented after new blood test breakthrough." http://www.telegraph.co.uk/news/science/science-news/ 10951689/Alzheimers-disease-could-be-prevented-after-new-blood-test-breakthrough.html.

Knapton, S. (2015) "Dementia research gets 13 times less funding than cancer, figures show." http://www.telegraph.co.uk/news/health/news/11532982/ Dementia-research-gets-13-times-less-funding-than-cancer-figures-show.html.

Koivisto, A.M., I. Hallikainen, T. Välimäki et al. (2016) "Early psychosocial intervention does not delay institutionalization in persons with mild Alzheimer disease and has impact on neither disease progression nor caregivers' well-being: ALSOVA 3-year follow-up." *International Journal of Geriatric Psychiatry* 31: 273–83.

Kontos, P., K.L. Miller, R. Colobong, L.I. Palma Lazgare et al. (2016) "Elder-clowning in long-term dementia care: Results of a pilot study." *Journal of the American Geriatrics Society* 64 (2): 347–53.

Kosik, K.S. and E. Clegg (2010) *The Alzheimer's Solution: How Today's Care is Failing Millions and How We Can Do Better.* Amherst, NY: Prometheus Books.

Kouwenhoven, P.S.C., N.J.H. Raijmakers, J.J.M. van Delden, J.A.C. Rietjens et al. (2015) "Opinions about euthanasia and advanced dementia: A qualitative study among Dutch physicians and members of the general public." *BMC Medical Ethics* 16: 7. http://www.biomedcentral.com/1472-6939/16/7.

Kuiper, J.S., M. Zuidersma, R.C. Oude Voshaar, S.U. Zuidema et al. (2015) "Social relationships and risk of dementia: A systematic review and meta-analysis of longitudinal cohort studies." *Ageing Research Reviews* 22: 39–57.

Kunkle, F. (2015) "Alzheimer's spurs the fearful to change their lives to delay it." *Washington Post.* https://www.washingtonpost.com/local/social-issues/fear-of-alzheimers-is-everywhere-but-its-spurring-some-people-to-change-their-lives-for-the-better/2015/07/04/c0600046-192a-11e5-93b7-5eddc056ad8a_story.html.

Lab Tests Online (2014) "Blood test shows very preliminary results in predicting Alzheimer disease." https://labtestsonline.org/news/140326alzheimer/.

Lai, C.K., J.H. Yeung, V. Mok and I. Chi (2009) "Special care units for dementia individuals with behavioural problems." *Cochrane Database Systems Review* 4: CD006470.

Lamm, R.D. and R.H. Blank (2007) *Condition Critical: A New Moral Vision for U.S. Health Care.* Golden, CO: Fulcrum Press.

Larson, E.B. and K.M. Langa (2017) "What's the "take home" from research on dementia trends." *PLoS Medicine* 14 (3): e1002236.

Larson, E.B., K. Yaffe, and K.M. Langa (2013) "New insights into the dementia epidemic." *New England Journal of Medicine* 369 (24): 2275–77.

Laxton, A.W. and A.M. Lozano (2013) "Deep brain stimulation for the treatment of Alzheimer's disease and dementias." *World Neurosurgery* 80 (3–4): S28.e1–S28.e8.

Laxton, A.W., D.F. Tang-Wai, M.P. McAndrews et al. (2010) "A phase 1 trial of deep brain stimulation of memory circuits in Alzheimer's disease." *Annals of Neurology* 68 (4): 521–34.

Le Couteur, D.G., B. Bateman and C. Brayne (2018) "Dalopirdine: Another disappointment for people with dementia." *British Medical Journal* 360: k753.

Lerner, A.J. (2013) "Amyloid imaging: The court of public opinion." *Neurology* 81: 1108–09.

Lewis, S.J. and S.R. Leeder (2009) "Why health reform?" *Medical Journal of Australia* 191 (5): 270–72.

Lichtner, V., D. Dowding, P. Esterhuizen, S. José Closs et al. (2014) "Pain assessment for people with dementia: A systematic review of systematic reviews of pain assessment tools." *BMC Geriatrics* 14: 138.

Lin, F.R. and M. Albert (2014) "Hearing loss and dementia—Who is listening?" *Aging Mental Health* 18: 671–73.

Lin, J.S., E. O'Connor, R. Rossom, L.A. Perdue et al. (2013) "Screening for cognitive impairment in older adults: An evidence update for the U.S. Preventive Services Task Force." Evidence Report No. 107. AHRQ Publication No. 14-05198-EF-1. Rockville, MD: Agency for Healthcare Research and Quality.

Lines, L.M., N.A. Sherif and J.M. Wiener (2014) *Racial and Ethnic Disparities among Individuals with Alzheimer's Disease in the United States: A Literature Review*. Research Triangle Park, NC: RTI Press.

Liu, Y., J.T Yu, H.F. Wang, P.R. Han et al. (2015) "APOE genotype and neuroimaging markers of Alzheimer's disease: Systematic review and meta-analysis." *Journal of Neurology and Neurosurgery Psychiatry* 86 (2): 127–34.

Livingston, G., J. Barber, P. Rapaport et al. (2014) "START (STrAtegies for RelaTives) study: A pragmatic randomised controlled trial to determine the clinical effectiveness and cost-effectiveness of a manual-based coping strategy programme in promoting the mental health of carers of people with dementia." *Health Technology Assessment* 18: 1–242.

Livingston, G., A. Sommerlad, V. Orgeta, S.G. Costafreda et al. (2017) "Dementia prevention, intervention, and care." *The Lancet.* https://doi.org/10.1016/S0140-6736(17)31363-6.

Loy, C.T., P.R. Schofield, A.M. Turner and J.B. Kwok (2014) "Genetics of dementia." *The Lancet* 383 (9919): 828–40.

Lozano, A.M., L. Fosdick, M.M. Chakravarty, J-M. Leoutsakos et al. (2016) "A phase II study of fornix deep brain stimulation in mild Alzheimer's disease." *Journal of Alzheimer's Disease* 54 (2): 777–87.

Luan, K., J.L. Rosales and K.Y. Lee (2013) "Viewpoint: Crosstalks between neurofibrillary tangles and amyloidplaque formation." *Ageing Research Review* 12: 174–181.

Luchsinger, J.A. (2010) "Diabetes, related conditions, and dementia." *Journal of the Neurological Sciences* 299 (1–2): 35–38.

Luengo-Fernandez, R., J. Leal and A. Gray (2015) "UK research spend in 2008 and 2012: Comparing stroke, cancer, coronary heart disease and dementia." *BMJ Open 2015*; 5: e006648. https://doi.org/10.1136/bmjopen-2014-006648.

Marceglia, S., S. Mrakic-Sposta, M. Rosa, R. Ferrucci, F. Mameli et al. (2016) "Transcranial direct current stimulation modulates cortical neuronal activity in Alzheimer's disease." *Frontiers in Neuroscience* 10: 134. https://doi.org/10.3389/fnins.2016.00134.

Mariani, E., M. Vernooij-Dassen, R. Koopmans, Y. Engels and R. Chattat (2017) "Shared decision-making in dementia care planning: Barriers and facilitators in two European countries." *Aging & Mental Health* 21 (1): 31–39.

Marmor, T.R., R. Freeman and K.G.H. Okma (2009) "Comparative policy analysis and health care: An introduction." In T.R. Marmor, R. Freeman and K.G.H. Okma, eds., *Comparative Studies and the Politics of Modern Medical Care.* New Haven, CT: Yale University Press.

Maslen, H., T. Douglas, R. Cohen Kadosh, N. Levy and J. Savulescu (2014) "The regulation of cognitive enhancement devices: Extending the medical model." *Journal of Law and the Biosciences* 1: 68–93.

Max Planck Institute for Human Development and Stanford Center on Longevity (2014) "A consensus on the brain training industry from the scientific community." http://longevity.stanford.edu/a-consensus-on-the-brain-training-industry-from-the-scientific-community-2/.

Mayeda, E.R., M.M. Glymour, C.P. Quesenberry and R.A. Whitmer (2014) "Inequalities in dementia incidence between six racial and ethnic groups over 14 years." *Alzheimer's & Dementia: The Journal of the Alzheimer's Association* 12 (3): 216–24.

Mazure, C.M. and J. Swendsen (2016) "Sex differences in Alzheimer's disease and other dementias." *Lancet Neurology* 15 (5): 451–52.

McCrae, N. (2014) "Assisted suicide and dementia." http://www.carenotkilling.org.uk/medical-opinion/assisted-suicide-and-dementia/.

McCrae, N. and J. Bloomfield (2013) "Mental health nursing and assisted dying." *Journal of Psychiatric & Mental Health Nursing* 20: 655–61.

Meiland, F., A. Innes, G. Mountain, L. Robinson, et al. (2017) "Technologies to support community-dwelling persons with dementia: A position paper on issues regarding development, usability, effectiveness and cost-effectiveness, deployment, and ethics." *JMIR Rehabilitation and Assistive Technologies* 4 (1): e1. https://doi.org/10.2196/rehab.6376.

Meinzer, M., R. Lindenberg, M.T. Phan, L. Ulm et al. (2015) "Transcranial direct current stimulation in mild cognitive impairment: Behavioral effects and neural mechanisms." *Alzheimer's and Dementia* 11 (9): 1032–40.

Meng, X. and C. D'Arcy (2012) "Education and dementia in the context of the cognitive reserve hypothesis: A systematic review with meta-analyses and qualitative analyses." *PLoS ONE* 7: e38268.

MetLife Mature Market Institute (2010) *The MetLife Study of Working Caregivers and Employer Health Care Costs.* Westport, CT: MetLife Mature Market Institute.

MetLife Mature Market Institute (2011) *The MetLife Study of Caregiving Costs to Working Caregivers: Double Jeopardy for Baby Boomers Caring for Their Parents.* Westport, CT: MetLife Mature Market Institute.

Mielke, M.M., P. Vemuri and W.A. Rocca (2014) "Clinical epidemiology of Alzheimer's disease: Assessing sex and gender differences." *Clinical Epidemiology* 6: 37–48.

Mielke, M.M., M.M. Machulda, C.E. Hagen, T.J. Christianson et al. (2016) "Influence of amyloid and APOE on cognitive performance in a late middle-aged cohort." *Alzheimer's and Dementia* 12 (3): 281–91.

Miller, F.G. and P.S. Appelbaum (2018) "Physician-assisted death for psychiatric patients—Misguided public policy." *New England Journal of Medicine* 378: 883–85.

Miller, D.G., R. Dresser and S.Y.H. Kim (2018) "Advance euthanasia directives: A controversial case and its ethical implications." *Journal of Medical Ethics.* https://doi.org/10.1136/medethics-2017-104644.

Moll van Charante, E.P., E. Richard, L.S. Eurelings, J.W. van Dalen et al. (2016) "Effectiveness of a 6-year multidomain vascular care intervention to prevent dementia (preDIVA): A cluster-randomised controlled trial." *Lancet* 388: 797–805.

Mordor Intelligence (2016) "Global Alzheimer's diagnosis and drugs market—Growth, trends and forecast (2016–2021)." http://www.mordorintelligence.com/industry-reports/alzheimers-diagnosisand-drugs-market.

Moyle, W. and S. O'Dwyer (2012) "Quality of life in people living with dementia in nursing homes." *Current Opinions in Psychiatry* 25: 480–84.

Mrakic-Sposta, S., M. Rosa, R. Ferrucci, F. Mameli et al. (2016) "Transcranial direct current stimulation modulates cortical neuronal activity in Alzheimer's disease." *Frontiers in Neuroscience* 10: 134. https://doi.org/10.3389/fnins.2016.00134.

Muramoto, O. (2010) "Socially and temporally extended end-of-life decision-making process for dementia patients." *Journal of Medical Ethics.* https://doi.org/10.1136/jme.2010.038950.

Nadash, P. and Y-C. Shih (2012) "Introducing social insurance for long-term care in Taiwan: Key issues." *International Journal of Social Welfare.* https://doi.org/10.1111/j.1468-2397.2011.00862.x.

Nakamura, A., N. Kaneko, V.L. Villemagne, T. Kato et al. (2018) "High performance plasma amyloid-β biomarkers for Alzheimer's disease." *Nature* 554: 249–54.

Napoletan, A. (2016) "Dementia care: What in the world is a dementia village?" http://www.alzheimers.net/2013-08-07/dementia-village/.

National Academies of Sciences, Engineering, and Medicine (NASEM) (2017) *Preventing Cognitive Decline and Dementia: A Way Forward.* Washington, DC: The National Academies Press.

National Association of State Units on Aging (2005) *Nursing Home Abuse Risk Prevention Profile and Checklist.* Washington, DC: National Center on Elder Abuse.

Naylor, M.D., L.H. Aiken, E.T. Kurtzman, D.M. Olds and K.B. Hirshman (2011) "The importance of transitional care in achieving health reform." *Health Affairs* 30 (4): 746–54.

Newport, M.T. (2011) *Alzheimer's Disease: What if There Was a Cure? The story of Ketones.* Laguna Beach, CA: Basic Health Publications.

Ng, T., C. Harrington, M. Musumeci and E.L. Reaves (2014) *Medicaid Home and Community-Based Services Programs: 2010 Data Update.* Washington, DC: Kaiser Family Foundation.

Norton, S., F.E. Matthews, D.E. Barnes, K. Yaffe and C. Brayne (2014) "Potential for primary prevention of Alzheimer's disease: An analysis of population-based data." *Lancet Neurology* 13: 788–94.

Novacic, I. (2016) "Alzheimer's patients test deep brain stimulation to help boost memory." http://www.cbsnews.com/news/for-alzheimers-patients-new-clinical-trial-could-help-stimulate-memory/.

Novella, S. (2015) "US Department of Justice goes after supplements." https://sciencebasedmedicine.org/us-department-of-justice-goes-after-supplements/.

Oizilbash, N., J. Gregson, M.E. Johnson, N. Pearce et al. (2015) "BMI and risk of dementia in two million people over two decades: A retrospective cohort study." *The Lancet: Diabetes and Endocrinology* 3 (6): 431–36.

Ontario Health Technology Assessment Commission (2013) "Vitamin B12 and cognitive function: An evidencebased analysis." *Ontario Health Technology Assessment Service* 13 (23): 1–45.

O'Rourke, H.M., W. Duggleby, K.D. Fraser and L. Jerke (2015) "Factors that affect quality of life from the perspective of people with dementia: A metasynthesis." *Journal of the American Geriatrics Society* 63 (1): 24–38.

Owen, J.E., K.T. Goode and W.E. Haley (2001) "End of life care and reactions to death in African-American and white family caregivers of relatives with Alzheimer's disease." *Omega (Westport)* 43: 349–61.

Owen, A.M., A. Hampshire, J.A. Grahn, R. Stenton, S. Dajani, A.S. Burns et al. (2010) "Putting brain training to the test." *Nature* 465 (7299): 775–78.

Palmour, N. and E. Racine (2011) "Direct-to-consumer marketing of dietary supplements for dementia: An example of unhealthy commerce of neuroscience." *AJOB Neuroscience* 2 (4): 30–33.

Panza, G.A., B.A. Taylor, H.V. MacDonald, B.T. Johnson et al. (2018) "Can exercise improve cognitive symptoms of Alzheimer's disease? A meta-analysis."

Journal of the American Geriatrics Society. https://doi.org/10.1111/jgs.15241.

Park, A-L. (2014) "Is there anything special about intergenerational approaches to older people with dementia? A review." *Journal of Alzheimer's Disease & Parkinsonism* 4: 172–80.

Pavolini, E. and H. Theobald (2015) "Long-term care policies." In E. Kuhlmann, R.H. Blank, I.L. Bourgeault and C. Wendt, eds., *The Palgrave International Handbook of Healthcare Policy and Governance.* Basingstoke: Palgrave, pp. 462–78.

PharmaFocus (2013) "Biomarkers in Alzheimer's disease." http://www.insightpharmareports.com/Affiliated-Reports/Global-Data/PharmaFocus--Biomarkers-in-Alzheimer-s-Disease/–.

Pinzon, L.C.E., M. Claus, K.M. Perrar, K.I. Zepf et al. (2013) "Dying with dementia: Symptom burden, quality of care, and place of death." *Deutsches Ärzteblatt International* 110: 195–202.

Porteri, C., E. Albanese, C. Scerri, M.C. Carrillo et al. (2017) "The biomarker-based diagnosis of Alzheimer's disease: Ethical and societal issues." *Neurobiology of Aging* 52: 132–40.

Power, G.A. (2010) *Dementia Beyond Drugs: Changing the Culture of Care.* Baltimore, MD: Health Professions Press, Inc.

Prince, M.J. (2017) "Progress on dementia—Leaving no one behind." *The Lancet.* https://doi.org/10.1016/S0140-6736(17)31757-9.

Prince, M.J., A. Wimo, M. Guerchet, G.C. Ali et al. (2015a) *World Alzheimer Report 2015: The Global Impact of Dementia: An Analysis of Prevalence, Incidence, Cost and Trends.* London: Alzheimer's Disease International.

Prince, M.J., F. Wu, Y. Guo, L.M. Gutierrez Robledo et al. (2015b) "The burden of disease in older people and implications for health policy and practice." *Lancet* 385: 549–62.

Prince, M.J., G.C. Ali, M. Guerchet, A.M. Prina et al. (2016) "Recent global trends in the prevalence and incidence of dementia, and survival with dementia." *Alzheimer's Research and Therapy* 8: 23. https://doi.org/10.1186/s13195-016-0188-8.

Prosporo, S. (2015) "A patient's decision: Dementia and euthanasia." https://sozoprosporo.com/2015/12/.

Rabins, P.V. (2007) "Can suicide be a rational and ethical act in persons with early or pre-dementia?" *American Journal of Bioethics* 7: 47–49.

Racine, E., H.A. van der Loos and J. Illes (2007) "Internet marketing of neuro-products: New practices and healthcare policy challenges." *Cambridge Quarterly of Healthcare Ethics* 16 (2): 181–94.

Rahimi, J. and G.G. Kovacs (2014) "Prevalence of mixed pathologies in the aging brain." *Alzheimer's Research and Therapy* 6 (9): 82–89.

Ramnarace, C. (2010) "The high costs of caring for Alzheimer's patients." http://www.aarp.org/relationships/caregiving/info-10-2010/the_high_costs_of_caring_for_alzheimers_patients.html.

Rapaport, P., G. Livingston, A. Mulla, J. Murray and C. Cooper (2017) "A systematic review of the effective components of psychosocial interventions delivered by care home staff to people with dementia." *BMJ Open* 7: e014177.

Rawlings, A.M., A.R. Sharrett, A.L.C. Schneider, J. Coresh, M. Albert et al. (2014) "Diabetes in midlife and cognitive change over 20 years: The Atherosclerosis Risk in Communities Neurocognitive Study." *Annals of Internal Medicine* 161 (11): 785–93.

Redfoot, D., L. Feinberg and A. Houser (2013) *The Aging of the Baby Boom and the Growing Care Gap: A Look at Future Declines in the Availability of Family Caregivers.* Washington, DC: AARP Public Policy Institute.

Redick, T.S., Z. Shipstead, T.L. Harrison, K.L. Hicks et al. (2013) "No evidence of intelligence improvement after working memory training: A randomized, placebo-controlled study." *Journal of Experimental Psychology: General* 142 (2): 359–79.

Reese, P.P., A.L. Caplan, R.D. Bloom, P.L. Abt and J.H. Karlawish (2010) "How should we use age to ration health care? Lessons from the case of kidney transplantation." *Journal of the American Geriatric Society* 58: 1980–86.

Reid, T.R. (2015) "Where's the war on Alzheimer's?" *AARP Bulletin* (Jan/Feb). http://www.aarp.org/health/brain-health/info-2015/alzheimers-research.html.

Reinhard, S.C., E. Kassner, A. Houser, K. Ujvari et al. (2014) "Raising expectations: A state scorecard on long-term services and supports for older adults, people with physical disabilities, and family caregivers." http://www.longtermscorecard.org/.

Research!America Health Poll (2006) "Top concerns about aging: Failing health, mental ability." http://www.researchamerica.org/sites/default/files/uploads/poll2006mentalhealth.pdf.

Ritchie, K., C.W. Ritchie, K. Yaffe, I. Skoog, and N. Scarmeas (2015) "Is late-onset Alzheimer's disease really a disease of midlife?" *Alzheimer's and Dementia: Translational Research and Clinical Interventions* 1 (2): 122–30.

Robbins, N.M. and J.L. Bernat (2017) "Should dementia be accepted as a disability to help restore hope during cognitive decline?" *AMA Journal of Ethics* 19 (7): 649–55.

Robinson, H., B. Macdonald, N. Kerse and E. Broadbent (2013) "The psychosocial effects of a companion robot: A randomized controlled trial." *Journal of the American Medical Directors Association* 14: 661–67.

Roth, M. (1996) "Euthanasia and related ethical issues in dementias of later life with special reference to Alzheimer's disease." *British Medical Bulletin* 52 (2): 63–79

Sabat, S.R. (2001) *The Experience of Alzheimer's Disease: Life Through a Tangled Veil.* Oxford, UK: Blackwell Publishers.

Sabat, S.R. (2008) "A bio-psycho-social approach to dementia." In M. Downs and B. Bowers, eds., *Excellence in Dementia Care: Research into Practice.* Maidenhead: Open University Press.

Sabat, S.R. (2018) *Alzheimer's Disease and Dementia: What Everyone Needs to Know.* Oxford: Oxford University Press.

Sachdev, P.S., D. Blacker, D.G. Blazer, M. Ganguli et al. (2014) "Classifying neurocognitive disorders: The DSM-5 approach." *Nature Reviews Neurology* 10: 634–42.

Sampson, E.L. (2010) "Palliative care for people with dementia." *British Medical Bulletin* 96: 159–74.

Satizabal, C.L., A.S. Beiser, V. Chouraki, G. Chêne et al. (2016) "Incidence of dementia over three decades in the Framingham Heart Study." *New England Journal of Medicine* 374: 523–32.

Sauer, A. (2016) "Benefits of deep brain stimulation for Alzheimer's." http://www.alzheimers.net/8-3-15-benefits-of-deep-brain-stimulation-for-alzheimers/.

SCAN Foundation (2013) "Who pays for long-term care in the U.S.?" Long Beach, CA: SCAN Foundation. http://www.thescanfoundation.org/who-pays-long-term-care-us.

Scheltens, P., T.W. Twisk, R. Blesa, E. Scarpini et al. (2012) "Efficacy of Souvenaid in mild Alzheimer's disease: Results from a randomized, controlled trial." *Journal of Alzheimer's Disease* 31: 225–36.

Schubert, C.C., M. Callahan, C.M. Perkins, A.J. Hui and H.C. Hendrie (2008) "Acute care utilization by dementia caregivers within urban primary care practices." *Journal of General Internal Medicine* 23 (11): 1736–40.

Schürks, M., R.J. Glynn, P.M. Rist, C. Tzourio and T. Kurth (2010) "Effects of vitamin E on stroke subtypes: Meta-analysis of randomised controlled trials." *British Medical Journal* 341: c5702.

Schwarzinger, M., B.G. Pollock, O.S.M. Hasan, C. Dufouil and J. Rehm (2018) "Contribution of alcohol use disorders to the burden of dementia in France 2008–13: A nationwide retrospective cohort study." *The Lancet Public Health.* https://doi.org/10.1016/S2468-2667(18)30022-7.

Searight, H.R. and J. Gafford (2005) "Cultural diversity at the end of life: Issues and guidelines for family physicians." *American Family Physician* 71 (3): 515–22.

Sharp, R. (2012) "The dangers of euthanasia and dementia: How Kantian thinking might be used to support non-voluntary euthanasia in cases of extreme dementia." *Bioethics* 26 (5): 231–35.

Shih, R.A., T.W. Concannon, J.L. Liu and E.M. Friedman (2014) "Improving dementia long-term care: A policy blueprint." *Rand Health Quarterly* 4 (2): 2.

Shrank, W.H., J.S. Kutner, T. Richardson, R.A. Mularski et al. (2005) "Focus group findings about the influences of communication preferences in end-of-life care." *Journal of General Internal Medicine* 2(8): 703–9.

Simons, D.J., W.R. Boot, N. Charness, S.E. Gathercole et al. (2016) "Do "brain-training" programs work?" *Psychological Science in the Public Interest* 17 (3): 103–86.

Sinclair, N. (2016) "The financial and emotional toll of America's Alzheimer's problem." http://finance.yahoo.com/news/alzheimers-most-expensive-disease-caregivers-cost-190758660.html;_ylt=A0LEV12541VYQZoAsQFXNyoA;_ylu=X3oDMTEyaTkzYXJyBGNvbG8DYmYxBHBvcwMxBHZ0aWQDQjMyMTlfMQRzZWMDc3I-.

Sinforiani, E., A. Citterio, C. Zucchella, G. Bono et al. (2010) "Impact of gender differences on the outcome of Alzheimer's disease." *Dementia* 30: 147–54.

Skinner, J.S., D.O. Staiger and E.S. Fisher (2006) "Is technological change in medicine always worth it? The case of myocardial infarction." *Health Affairs* 25: w34–w47.

Smith, W.J. (2013) "Swiss suicide clinic kills Alzheimer's patient, euthanasia activists applaud." http://www.lifenews.com/2013/06/09/swiss-suicide-clinic-kills-alzheimers-patient-euthanasia-activists-applaud/

Smith, M., K.C. Buckwalter, H. Kang, V. Ellingrod and S.K. Schultz (2008) "Dementia-specific assisted living: Clinical factors and psychotropic medication use." *Journal of the American Psychiatric Nurses Association* 14: 39–49.

Smith, A.D., S.M. Smith, C.A. de Jager et al. (2010) "Homocysteine-lowering by B vitamins slows the rate of accelerated brain atrophy in mild cognitive impairment: A randomized controlled trial." *PLoS ONE* 5: e12244.

Sofi, F., D. Valecchi, D. Bacci et al. (2011) "Physical activity and risk of cognitive decline: A meta-analysis of prospective studies." *Journal of Internal Medicine* 269: 107–17.

Sommerlad, A., J. Ruegger, A. Singh-Manoux, G. Lewis and G. Livingston (2017) "Marriage and risk of dementia: Systematic review and meta-analysis of observational studies." *Journal of Neurology, Neurosurgery and Psychiatry.* https://doi.org/10.1136/jnnp-2017-316274.

Spillman, B.C. and S.K. Long (2009) "Does high caregiver stress predict nursing home entry?" *Inquiry* 46: 140–61.

Sprung, C.L., P. Maia, H-H. Bulow, B. Ricou et al. (2007) "The importance of religious affiliation and culture on end-of-life decisions in European intensive care units." *Intensive Care Medicine* 33 (10): 1732–39.

Stem Cell Therapy Plus (2016) http://www.stemcelltherapyplus.com/.

StemGenex (2016) "Can stem cell therapy help patients with Alzheimer's disease?" https://stemgenex.com/studies/alzheimers-stem-cell-studies/?utm_source=bing&utm_medium=cpc&utm_campaign=Alzheimer%27s&utm_content=Stem%20Cell&utm_term=%2Balzheimers%20%2BStem%20%2BCell.

Stetka, B. (2016) "Reviving memory with an electrical current." http://www.npr.org/sections/health-shots/2016/05/14/477934952/can-electricity-be-used-to-treat-alzheimer-s-diseaseHealthNewsFromNPR.

Stites, S.D, J. Karlawish, K. Harkins, J.D. Rubright and D. Wolk (2017) "Awareness of mild cognitive impairment and mild Alzheimer's disease dementia diagnoses associated with lower self-ratings of quality of life in older adults." *The Journals of Gerontology, Series B: Psychological Sciences and Social Science.* https://doi. org/10.1093/geronb/gbx100.

Suehs, B.T., C.D. Davis, J. Alvir, D. van Amerongen et al. (2013) "The clinical and economic burden of newly diagnosed Alzheimer's disease in a medicare advantage population." *American Journal of Alzheimer's Disease and Other Dementias* 28 (4): 384–92.

Sulzer, J., S. Haller, F. Scharnowski, N. Weiskopf et al. (2013) "Real-time fMRI neurofeedback: Progress and challenges." *Neuroimage* 76: 386–99.

Sundström, A., O. Westerlund and E. Kotyrlo (2016) "Marital status and risk of dementia: A nationwide population-based prospective study from Sweden." *BMJ Open* 6: e008565.

Swan, G.E. and C.N. Lessov-Schlaggar (2007) "The effects of tobacco smoke and nicotine on cognition and the brain." *Neuropsychological Review* 17: 259–73.

Telegraph (2014) "Older people are more scared of dementia than cancer, poll finds." http://www.telegraph.co.uk/news/health/elder/11008905/Older-people-are-more-scared-of-dementia-than-cancer-poll-finds.html.

ten Brinke, L.F., N. Bolandzadeh, L.S. Nagamatsu, C.L. Hsu et al. (2017) "Aerobic exercise increases hippocampal volume in older women with probable mild cognitive impairment: A 6-month randomised controlled trial." *British Journal of Sports Medicine* 49 (4): https://doi.org/10.1136/bjsports-2013-093184.

The Thought Zone (2017) "The cure to dementia: A beverage?" https://mbman. wordpress.com/2017/06/01/the-cure-to-dementia-a-beverage/.

Theobald, H. and S. Hampel (2013) "Radical institutional change and incremental transformation: Long-term care insurance in Germany." In C. Ranci and E. Pavolini, eds., *Reforms in Long-term Care Policies in Europe.* Heidelberg and New York: Springer, pp. 117–38.

Theobald, H. and E. Ozanne (2016) "Multi-level governance and its effects in long-term care policies." In C. Gori, J-L. Fernández and R. Wittenberg, eds., *Long-term Care Reforms in OECD Countries: Successes and Failures.* Bristol: Policy Press, pp. 271–92.

Thomas, L.G. (1974) *The Lives of a Cell.* New York: Viking Press.

Thraves, L. (2015) "Stem cell research." https://www.alzheimers.org.uk/site/scripts/documents_info.php?documentID=430.

Tomlinson, E. and J. Stott (2014) "Assisted dying in dementia: A systematic review of the international literature on the attitudes of health professionals, patients, carers and the public, and the factors associated with these." *International Journal of Geriatric Psychiatry* 30 (1): 10–20.

Toms, G.R., C. Quinn, D.E. Anderson and L. Clare (2015) "Help yourself perspectives on self-management from people with dementia and their caregivers." *Qualitative Health Research* 25 (1): 87–98.

Topiwala, A, C.L. Allan, V. Valkanova et al. (2017) "Moderate alcohol consumption as risk factor for adverse brain outcomes and cognitive decline: Longitudinal cohort study." *British Medical Journal* 357: j2353.

Trafton, A. (2012) "In clinical trial, mixture developed at MIT appears to help overcome loss of connections between brain cells. Nutrient mixture improves memory in patients with early Alzheimer's." *MIT News.* http://news.mit.edu/2012/alzheimers-nutrient-mixture-0709.

University Health Network (UHN) (2016) "Deep brain stimulation continues to show promise for patients with mild Alzheimer's disease." *ScienceDaily.* www.sciencedaily.com/releases/2016/07/160719144831.htm.

van der Steen, J.T. (2010) "Dying with dementia: What we know after more than a decade of research." *Journal of Alzheimer's Disease* 22: 37–55.

van der Steen, J.T., I. Meuleman-Peperkamp and M.W. Ribbe (2009) "Trends in treatment of pneumonia among Dutch nursing home patients with dementia." *Journal of Palliative Medicine* 12: 789–95.

Veech, R.L. (2004) "The therapeutic implications of ketone bodies: The effects of ketone bodies in pathological conditions: Ketosis, ketogenic diet, redox states, insulin resistance, and mitochondrial metabolism." *Prostaglandins, Leukotrienes and Essential Fatty Acids* 70 (3): 309–19.

Verbeek, H., E. van Rossum, S.M. Zwakhalen, G.I. Kempen and J.P. Hamers (2009) "Small, homelike care environments for older people with dementia: A literature review." *International Psychogeriatrics* 21: 252–64.

Villemagne, V.L., W.E. Klunk, C.A. Mathis, C.C. Rowe et al. (2012) "Aβ Imaging: Feasible, pertinent, and vital to progress in Alzheimer's disease." *European Journal of Nuclear Medicine and Molecular Imaging* 39: 209–19.

Wada, T., H. Imai, E. Fukutomi et al. (2014) "Preferred feeding methods for dysphagia due to end-stage dementia in community-dwelling elderly people in Japan." *Journal of the American Geriatric Society* 62: 1810–11.

Wakabayashi, C. and K.M. Donato (2006) "Does caregiving increase poverty among women in later life? Evidence from the Health and Retirement Survey." *Journal of Health and Social Behavior* 47 (3): 258–74.

Ward A, S. Tardiff, C. Dye and H.M. Arrighi (2013) "Rate of conversion from prodromal Alzheimer's disease to Alzheimer's dementia: A systematic review of the literature." *Dementia and Geriatrics Cognitive Disorders Extra* 3: 320–32.

Weuve, J., L.E. Hebert, P.A. Scherr and D.A. Evans (2014) "Deaths in the United States among persons with Alzheimer's disease, 2010–2050." *Alzheimer's and Dementia* 10: e40–e46.

Wheeler, M. (2014) "Small trial by UCLA and Buck Institute succeeds using 'systems approach' to memory disorders: Memory loss associated with Alzheimer's reversed for first time." http://newsroom.ucla.edu/releases/memory-loss-associated-with-alzheimers-reversed-for-first-time.

Whitehouse, P.J. (2014) "The end of Alzheimer's disease—From biochemical pharmacology to ecopsychosociology: A personal perspective." *Biochemical Pharmacology* 88 (4): 677–81.

Whitehouse, P.J. and D. George (2008) *The Myth of Alzheimer's.* New York: St. Martin's Press.

Wiersma, E.C. and A. Denton (2016) "From social network to safety net: Dementia-friendly communities in rural Northern Ontario." *Dementia* 15 (1): 51–68.

Williams, B.O. (2000) "Ageism helps to ration medical treatment." *Health Bulletin* 58 (3): 198–202.

Williams, N., C. Dunford, A. Knowles and J. Warner (2007) "Public attitudes to life-sustaining treatments and euthanasia in dementia." *International Journal of Geriatric Psychiatry* 22: 1229–34.

Wimo, A. and M. Prince (2010) *World Alzheimer Report 2010: The Global Economic Impact of Dementia.* London: Alzheimer's Disease International.

Winblad, B., P. Amouyel, S. Andrieu, C. Ballard et al. (2016) "Defeating Alzheimer's disease and other dementias: A priority for European science and society." *Lancet Neurology* 15: 455–532.

Wise, J. (2018) "Large study is 'robust' evidence of link between chronic heavy drinking and dementia." *British Medical Journal* 360: k814.

Wolff, J. L., J. Feder and R. Schulz (2016) "Supporting family caregivers of older Americans." *New England Journal of Medicine* 375 (26): 2513–15.

Woods, B., E. Aguirre, A.E. Spector and M. Orrell (2012) "Cognitive stimulation to improve cognitive functioning in people with dementia." *Cochrane Database System Review* 2: CD005562.

Woolham, J. (2005) *Safe at Home: The Effectiveness of Assistive Technology in Supporting the Independence of People with Dementia: The Safe at Home Project.* London: Hawker Press.

WHO (2012) *Dementia: A Public Health Priority.* Geneva: WHO.

WHO (2015) "Governments commit to advancements in dementia research and care." http://www.who.int/mediacentre/news/releases/2015/action-on-dementia/en/.

WHO (2016) "WHO health statistics and information systems: Estimates for 2000–2012." http://www.who.int/healthinfo/global_burden_disease/estimates/en/index1.html.

WHO (2017a) Draft global action plan on the public health response to dementia. Report by the Director-General. April 3. http://apps.who.int/gb/ebwha/pdf_files/WHA70/A70_28-en.pdf?ua=1 (Accessed June 26, 2017).

WHO (2017b) "Seventieth World Health Assembly update, 29 May 2017." http://www.who.int/mediacentre/news/releases/2017/dementia-immunization-refuguees/en/.

WHO (2017c) "The global dementia observatory." http://www.who.int/mental_health/neurology/dementia/GDO/en/.

WHO (2017d) "The global health data observatory." http://apps.who.int/gho/data/node.home.

Wu, T-Y., C-P. Chen and T-R. Jinn (2011) "Traditional Chinese medicines and Alzheimer's disease." *Taiwanese Journal of Obstetrics & Gynecology* 50: e131–e135.

Xing, Y., Y. Tang and J. Jia (2015) "Sex differences in neuropsychiatric symptoms of Alzheimer's disease: The modifying effect of apolipoprotein E ε4 status." *Behavioural Neurology*. Published online October 11. https://doi.org/10.1155/2015/275256.

Yaffe, K., C. Falvey, T.B. Harris, A. Newman et al. (2013) "Effect of socioeconomic disparities on incidence of dementia among biracial older adults: Prospective study." *British Medical Journal* 347: f7051.

Yang, Z. and A. Levey (2015) "Gender differences: A lifetime analysis of the economic burden of Alzheimer's disease." *Women's Health Issues* 25 (5): 436–40.

Yang Y-H., C-L. Hsu, M.C. Chou, M. Kasai, et al. (2015) "Early symptoms of Alzheimer's disease in Japan and Taiwan." *Geriatrics and Gerontology International* 16 (7):797–803.

Young, J., M. Angevaren, J. Rusted and N. Tabet (2015) "Aerobic exercise to improve cognitive function in older people without known cognitive impairment." *Cochrane Database System Review* 4: CD005381.

Yuan, H., S. Tabarak, Jing Yu and Xu Lei (2015) "Transcranial direct current stimulation in patients with Alzheimer's disease: Challenges and responses." *ADMET & DMPK* 3 (3): 235–41.

Zakaib, G.D. (2016) "Souvenaid trial missed primary, partially met secondary endpoints." http://www.alzforum.org/news/conference-coverage/souvenaid-trial-missed-primary-partially-met-secondary-endpoints.

Zick, C.D., C.J. Mathews, J.S. Roberts, R. Cook-Deegan et al. (2005) "Genetic testing for Alzheimer's disease and its impact on insurance purchasing behavior." *Health Affairs* 24 (2): 483–90.

Zimmerman, S., W.L. Anderson, S. Brode et al. (2013) "Systematic review: Effective characteristics of nursing homes and other residential long-term care settings for people with dementia." *Journal of the American Geriatrics Society* 61: 1399–409.